Pra

Unhackable Moms of Addicted Loved Ones

As someone who works with people in jails and prisons, I know how important it is for families to understand addiction and how their actions affect their loved one's rehabilitation. Michelle shows moms how to love with boundaries, which is key to addiction recovery.

—Cat Hoke
Author of *A Second Chance: For You, For Me, and For the Rest of Us*
Speaker, Creator of Hustle 2.0, a self-directed, in-cell study program for incarcerated people, Defy Ventures, and Prison Entrepreneurship Program. In eighteen years, 11,000+ incarcerated people have graduated from her programs. Her efforts have led 7,000 executives, entrepreneurs, and investors to volunteer as mentors and employers. The programs reduce violence and have produced industry-leading recidivism rates of less than eight percent.

When your child is struggling with an addiction, everyone tells you to "focus on your own recovery" and says, "You need to take care of yourself." You know this is good advice, but it feels impossible when you're drowning in fear, grief, and frustration. *Unhackable Moms of Addicted Loved Ones* puts you back in the driver's seat of your own life. Michelle Weidenbenner calls on her experience to create a road map for other parents desperately searching for answers. Change and hope are on the horizon.

—Amber Hollingsworth, LPC, MAC
Owner, Founder, and Counselor at Hope for Families
Host of *Put the Shovel Down* on YouTube.com

Unhackable Moms of Addicted Loved Ones is a simple yet powerful thirty-day process for all moms of addicted loved ones to follow. Michelle shares her own experience, strength, and hope alongside powerful tools to guide moms on their healing journey. I'm grateful this book exists.

—Jesse Harless
Author of #1 best-selling book, *If Not You, Then Who?*
Jesse is a leader in the addiction recovery and mental health space. His passion is to help individuals and purpose-driven organizations share their voices to co-create a better world for all.

Unhackable Moms of Addicted Loved Ones is not your typical self-help book. It is Michelle's heartfelt invitation to start embodying your divine destiny. If you are the mother of an addicted loved one, you are sure to find the inspiration you need to begin your own healing journey. The tips, exercises, and reflection questions will empower you in unexpected ways. You will learn to honor your values, set healthy boundaries, and detach with love. Thank you, Michelle, for this magnificent gift.

—**Isabelle Wettergren**
Professional Recovery Coach
National Board-Certified Health and Wellness Coach
Mental Health Ambassador

If you are sick and tired of being sick and tired *Unhackable Moms* is just what you need. It is a powerful read. Get ready for change. With SUD (substance use disorder) affecting every family in America, it gives practical, applicable steps for a thirty-day plan to rewire one's thinking. Weidenbenner shares all perspectives, the user, the parents, the family, and friends. This book will open your eyes to how to stop being the victim and become the victor of your life. Join the movement Unhackable Moms.

—**Crystal Waltman**
Author of *Quitting to Win* , best-selling health book of the year

As a mom of someone who struggles with substance use disorder, I was drawn to Michelle because of her compassion and empathy toward those who suffer from addiction. As I got to know her, I learned that she was a person with great knowledge, strength, and determination for living life with intention. Michelle is passionate about helping women overcome their struggles so they can regain their life. If you are the mother affected by someone with an addiction, you will gain insight, wisdom, and most importantly, hope as you read this inspirational book.

—**Pam Lanhart**
Family Addiction Recovery Coach
Founder and Director of Thrive Family Recovery Resources
Author of *Praying Our Loved One Home*

This book teaches moms of addicted loved ones how to lead from within so they can take charge of their lives.

—**Linda Sue Key**
Addiction Specialist and Recovery Coach

UNHACKABLE MOMS OF ADDICTED LOVED ONES

Closing the Gap Between Havoc and Hope

Other Books by Michelle Weidenbenner

*Moms Letting Go Without Giving Up, Seven Steps to
Self-Recovery
Fractured Not Broken
Scattered Links
Cache a Predator
The Éclair series
Wily and the Canine Pandemic
Glow Girl*

UNHACKABLE MOMS OF ADDICTED LOVED ONES

Closing the Gap Between Havoc and Hope

The 30-Day Program That Empowers You to
Cope with Chaos, Balance Bold Boundaries,
and Listen without Lecturing

MICHELLE WEIDENBENNER

Inspired by *Unhackable*
The Wall Street Journal and *USA Today* Best Seller
by Kary Oberbrunner

Library of Congress Control Number: 2022904266
Paperback ISBN: 978-1-955164-09-2
Hardback ISBN: 978-1-955164-10-8
Ebook ISBN: 978-1-955164-11-5
Available in hardcover, softcover, e-book, and audiobook.

To protect the privacy of those who shared their stories with the author, some details and names have been changed. Any internet addresses (websites, blogs, etc.) and telephone numbers printed in this book are offered as a resource. They are not in any way intended to be or imply an endorsement by Unhackable Press, nor does Unhackable Press vouch for the content of these sites and numbers for the life of this book.

Disclaimer: The information provided in this book is intended for your general knowledge and support and is not a substitute for profession medical advice or treatment for medical conditions and/or advice/guidance by professionals with expertise, such as a counselor, physician, or addiction professional. You assume full responsibility for how you choose to use this information. You should not use this information to diagnose or treat a health problem or disease without consulting with a qualified healthcare provider or expert. Always seek the advice of a physician or other qualified healthcare provider or expert before making any decisions about your health care options.

Scripture quotations marked (NRSV) are taken from the New Revised Standard Version Bible (NRSV), copyright © 1989 the Division of Christian Education of the National Council of the Churches of Christ in the United States of America. Used by permission. All rights reserved worldwide.

Scripture quotations marked (NIV) are taken from the Holy Bible, New International Version®, NIV®. Copyright © 1973, 1978, 1984, 2011 by Biblica, Inc.™ Used by permission of Zondervan. All rights reserved worldwide. www.zondervan.comThe "NIV" and "New International Version" are trademarks registered in the United States Patent and Trademark Office by Biblica, Inc.™

Dedicated to
Children who died with a substance use disorder,
feeling shamed, invisible, and misunderstood.
Your lives mattered.

Children born into circumstances that left
them vulnerable and victims of trauma.
We are listening.

Moms of addicted loved ones who grieve the loss of dreams
they have for their addicted and incarcerated children.
You are not alone.

Moms who want to heal so they may recapture
their identity and purpose to reach their dreams.
Let's do this together.

Moms who want to join the movement
to stop the addiction epidemic.
We can do great things together.
Join us!

Contents

Part One: Unveiling

Part Two: Flawless Hope Anatomy

Part Three: Deliberate Mom Focus

Part Four: Optimal Mom Performance

Part Five: The Boon Ceremony

Appendices

Foreword

When Michelle decided to write *Unhackable Moms of Addicted Loved Ones*, I knew she was the perfect person to bring hope and healing to hurting moms. Michelle has a heart of gold. She's an incredible leader and a total giver. She is passionate about helping moms recover so they can have the energy to fight this epidemic.

Like many other moms, Michelle endured years of uncertainty while her son and daughter-in-law suffered from a substance use disorder (SUD). She often feared they would die of an overdose and leave their children parentless. Thankfully, today they are three years sober and in recovery.

The more Michelle learned about SUDs, the more she realized what she didn't know and wondered how many other moms needed to know what she was learning. She knew how important it was for other moms to share, learn, and heal together too. She thought, *I can't make a dent in this epidemic, but if I empower one million moms of addicted loved ones to find peace, then together we can make a difference.*

Michelle understood that when moms recover from the havoc, they become hope builders for their children. That's why, in this thirty-day program, she inspires moms to break free from worry so they can reach their full potential as God's creation. Using the tools and hope Michelle offers, moms will identify their culprit, plan boundaries, find empathy, choose peace, dump the shame, and jump for joy as they focus on recapturing their identity and purpose.

If you're committed to fighting this disease for the sake of your children and the generations to follow, read this book and join the All-Mighty Mom Movement today!

—Kary Oberbrunner
Wall Street Journal and *USA Today* bestselling author
CEO of Igniting Souls Publishing Agency

A Note to You, The Reader

Nobody gets out of this world alive. We all will die, which is why we must live a full life while we can.

For me, living a full life means living with purpose and helping build God's kingdom using my gifts and talents. When I get stuck, I don't live in my purpose.

Before I started advocating for moms of addicted loved ones (ALO), I enjoyed a life of retirement. I spent my free time writing fiction, and it was a blast. When addiction hacked my family, I froze. My productivity stopped.

It took me a while to understand addiction as a disease and learn how to help my family, but once I did, I felt called to help others—like you—who might be hacked in a similar way. My prayer is that, through this book, God will use me to help lead you into your purpose.

Addiction is a spiritual battle. Faith has helped me cope and brought me hope. Fighting addiction and serving moms of addicted loved ones improved my relationship with God. I share my spiritual beliefs with you, hoping you'll respect them, as I respect your beliefs and understand they might be different from mine.

To keep things simple, I use the gender reference *he* throughout the book, even though many women struggle with a substance use disorder too.

I call myself the Chief Hope Builder. In this book, if you'll allow me, I'll position myself as your coach and hope builder, not to preach or cast judgment, but to cheer for you to become Unhackable. Why? Because you and your child are worth the fight. God is counting on you to use your gifts to build His kingdom. But you can't give what you don't have, and if you don't have hope, you can't give it to others.

The addiction landscape is ugly. Though the stigma is lifting, we still have a long way to go. The disorder leads to homelessness, hopelessness, and accidental overdoses. It fills our jails and prisons. Rehab options are expensive, and some aren't led by physicians who treat dual diagnoses. Some rehabs don't employ trauma experts. Many of our loved ones can't afford evidence-based rehabilitation centers. Much work needs done, and who better to help fight this cause than you—a mom who understands the physical, spiritual, emotional, and financial cost of this disease?

I implore you to embrace this thirty-day program so you can break free from the shame, guilt, and blame that hold you back from living a purposeful life. The world needs the energy of your skills and gifts to improve the addiction landscape.

—Michelle Weidenbenner
Founder of Chief Hope Builders, Moms Letting Go,
and the All-Mighty Mom Tribe

Meet the All-Mighty Mom Tribe Contributors

Below are a few moms from the All-Mighty Mom Tribe who have courageously and generously shared parts of their stories in this book. They, as I do, believe that healing happens in communities. When I opened the subscription membership to the All-Mighty Mom Tribe, it was to help moms heal together. I did it to unite moms so they wouldn't feel alone. What I didn't expect was the inspiration, healing, and transformation these women would bring to my faith life.

Sandy

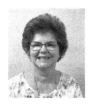 Christian wife and mom of three—a daughter in heaven and two sons, one recovering from an SUD—Sandy is a retired family and consumer science teacher and guidance counselor. She is also a quilter, seamstress, knitter, and chief encourager. An articulate, life-long learner, Sandy is compassionate, faithful, loyal, spiritual, and committed to helping moms on this journey.

Lucretia

Wife to the same man for forty-three years and mom to seven—one a recovering loved one—Lucretia is Christ-passionate, thoughtful, and inspirational. As a speaker and a life coach, Lucretia leads Bible studies and coaches moms who have addicted and incarcerated loved ones. She is a loyal friend.

Brooke

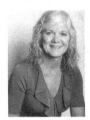

Mom to two sons—one a recovering loved one—Brooke is trustworthy, dependable, resilient, caring, passionate, and a dog lover. Brooke leads "Write, Read, and Listen," a journaling and sharing exercise in our support groups. She is faithful and generous.

Colleen

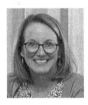

Mom of a recovering son and two daughters. NayNay to seven. Colleen is funny, kind, giving, thoughtful, and able to see the good in others. Her love for the elderly shines with empathetic patience and compassion.

Teresa

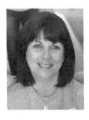

Mother to two recovering loved ones, Teresa is faithful, trustworthy, loving, and kind. Teresa is a strong supporter of compassionate care for homeless individuals and determined to never lose hope.

Darra

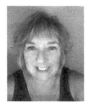 A widow who is parenting two special-needs grandchildren because of her daughter's substance use disorder, Darra is a Christ-centered encourager and prayer warrior. She is also a pickleball enthusiast.

PART ONE

Unveiling

DAY 1

Write Your Story

*The greatest burden a child must bear
is the unlived life of its parents.*

—Carl Jung

I sat on the end of the exam table during my annual physical. "Are you still taking vitamin D?" my doctor asked.

"Oh, no. I forgot."

"I don't understand," she said. "Take one every morning with breakfast. Why is that difficult?"

"There's so much going on in the morning. Sometimes I forget to eat."

She paused. "You forget to eat?"

I stared out the window. "My granddaughters live with me. Their parents are in the throes of addiction. Raising children at sixty is difficult, especially when I see how sick their parents have become. They might die."

"You have to take care of yourself, Michelle. Stress can cause life-threatening health issues."

3

I knew she spoke truth, but I also knew I couldn't control my anxiety. I wanted to stay calm and believe everything was going to turn out okay. But with more than 150 people dying of overdoses each day[1], I worried my son and daughter-in-law would be next.

At that moment, I didn't have faith. I couldn't breathe much less remember to take a vitamin.

My husband and I had looked forward to retirement; however, reentering a life of parenting hadn't been in the plans. Sleep eluded me, and my heart raced. My husband's disappointment made him crabby.

I knew I had to be strong and healthy for my grandchildren. They needed me. Their health would suffer if I didn't make myself a priority. Who else would make sure they didn't take responsibility for their parents' addiction? I had to show them their lives matter and they are loved; but wow, being responsible for them took energy.

The pressure of knowing how much my granddaughters needed me took my breath away and gave me palpitations. I often had thoughts like, *What if I die? Who will they have?*

With my doctor's help, I found the strength and courage to work on myself. I couldn't control my son's actions, but I could steer my life and choose the way I responded to him. Learning how wasn't easy. I couldn't relate to him. I didn't recognize the person he had become. His addiction had made him thin, jittery, unassertive, and unable to look me in the eye.

Unfortunately, I saw a very similar reflection when I looked in the mirror. I needed a healthy-living plan too. Who was I to judge him, wishing he would get into recovery, when I needed the same thing?

That day marked the beginning of my recovery, and my plan to help other moms began to take shape.

The Hacking Started Earlier

After the birth of my son, Ryan, my mom and dad came to see me for a few days. When they prepared to leave, I cried. I said to my mom, "I don't know what to do. I've never done this before."

"You'll figure it out. You're doing fine," she said. "You had five brothers. You can handle this."

I had never felt so alone. I'd only been married a year, and already I'd quit my job, left my hometown, and moved to a new community. There was no one to help.

Somehow, I managed. I read books on infant stages, joined the La Leche League to learn how to breastfeed, and intentionally set out to meet other moms with newborns.

As my son grew, so did I. Along the way, I learned that society depicts moms as women who nurture. We aren't told to stop nurturing and mothering our children when they become adults.

We're the ones who give them life and sustain it when they're infants, toddlers, and children. No wonder moms try to save and fix their addicted loved ones (ALOs). It's an innate part of our mother-DNA to rescue them. Moms feel their job description includes knowing how to love, parent, and be everything to their children, no matter how old they are, so it's understandable we learn to do too much for them.

From the first moment we saw our children, we nurtured each of them as best we could. We held them when they cried, we listened when they were bullied, and we skipped and jumped with them at the playground. We envisioned them as successful adults, and throughout their lives, we taught them to be independent and responsible.

As Ryan grew from infant to toddler and then progressed through his school years, I had dreams for him. I thought he'd have his own business one day.

What about you? What dreams did you have for your son or daughter when they were young?

Many moms get so focused on their children's lives they forget themselves. Some take part-time, low-paying jobs so they can be available for their families. Others stay home to care for their children. In between the babies and the bills, they forget themselves—who they are, what excites them, and what their passions are.

Our lives get hacked by mothering responsibilities. Once our children leave home, many of us don't know what to do with our lives. We don't know where we fit in. After spending years catering to our kids, we finally have time to ourselves, but we can't remember what we liked to do or what we wanted to accomplish.

Did that happen to you?

Were you distracted from achieving your life goal? Did you set aside your dream while you raised your children?

Unfulfilled dreams weigh heavy, but often moms feel selfish making themselves a priority. We think, *Good moms think of others first. The best moms put their children's needs first. What kind of mom would I be if I let my child struggle?*

If you've had those thoughts, you're not alone. Maybe you imagined a season for more *you time* after your children were grown, but one child developed an SUD, and you became stuck again. Now you think, *How can I let my child live on the streets and go hungry?*

To help your child, you become addicted to supporting them in unhealthy ways. Meanwhile, your dreams seem unimportant because you can't see past helping your child.

I'm here to tell you your dreams are important. Happiness might seem impossible when your child is ill, but with help, you will discover that when you get well, your child will find hope in your transformation, and he or she will want what you have.

I've heard it said that a mom is only as happy as her least happy child, but I disagree. It doesn't have to be this way. Happiness is a choice. Moms can find happiness despite their children's suffering. No, we don't want them to hurt, but we must find control in our lives when their actions are out of our control. We can learn to be Unhackable Moms of Addicted Loved Ones.

If we keep getting sidelined and sabotaged, we'll remain in an endless cycle of angst. Scrolling the latest newsfeed or social media channel won't silence our ache. Checking on our children multiple times a day isn't the way to focus on us or find peace either.

Each of us is hardwired to dream and do. This includes big dreams like building a house, completing a degree, or finishing a screenplay. It also includes small goals like running three times a week, organizing your closet, or planning your weekly meals.

When you know your daily goals and make progress, you feel good. When you get hacked by worrying about your addicted loved one, you feel mental and emotional anguish. If getting hacked becomes a pattern, you'll drift toward depression, emotional eating, or other unhealthy coping mechanisms. I've seen it happen.

Unfortunately, moms get hacked all the time. We fail to implement our ideas. We go from ideation to frustration or stagnation. Instead of embodying our divine destiny, we settle for a depraved reality and havoc. In the end, this hurts our children because they see their hopeless parents with unfulfilled dreams.

You were meant for more. But if you are like many other moms of addicted loved ones, you may not see the path toward *more* right now. As Chief Hope Builder, my goal for this book and my prayer for you is that what you discover about yourself in the next thirty days will empower you to find or rediscover your dreams and map out the path to making them come true.

Get Ready

Right now, you're minutes away from getting hacked. I'm not referring to your computer, phone, or bank account. Those types of hacks can be remedied. I'm referring to a hack costlier than all those combined.

I'm referring to your brain.

Have you ever had an amazing idea? If you're like most moms with addicted children, you started out excited, ready to make your dream come true. But then, your child started using, and your life changed. Your focus shifted to your child's problem. Nothing else mattered. You and your idea got sidelined. If so, you're not alone.

Hacking simply means someone or something gained unauthorized access. Although we often think of electronic devices getting hacked, humans become hacked too. Our bodies are composed of systems (respiratory, circulatory, digestive, and immune, to name a few), and our brains operate like supercomputers.

Navigating this noisy world long enough to accomplish daily tasks—much less accomplish our dreams—is nearly impossible, especially these days. The odds are clearly stacked against us, and temptations lurk less than an arm's length away—even with people who aren't dealing with an addiction crisis:

- **Smartphones hack us:** Statistics vary, but according to a study performed by dscout, on average people touch their phones 2,617 times a day.[2] (Heavy users touch 5,427 times. There were no statistics on how many times moms of addicted loved ones touch their phones, but I've talked with many who sleep with them turned on and next to them in bed, waiting for the call. The call that informs them their child has overdosed.)

- **Multitasking hacks us:** Multitasking is a myth. The brain can only do one cognitive activity at a time. Multitasking, more properly understood as switch-tasking, decreases productivity by up to 40 percent. According to Forbes, "Multitasking with electronic media caused a greater decrease in IQ than smoking pot."[3]

- **Social media hacks us:** Americans spend more than two hours a day on social media, with most of that time in small, unplanned bits of time that interrupt their work or other scheduled activities.

- **Streaming videos hack us:** According to ReelnReel, people spend eleven billion hours watching videos on Netflix every month.[4]

- **Advertisements hack us:** *The New York Times* reveals the average person sees 5,000 ads a day.[5]

- **Decision fatigue hacks us:** Researchers at Cornell University discovered the average person makes 226.7 food decisions a day.[6] This doesn't consider the 25,000 other decisions the average person makes daily. Moms with addicted children obsessively think about what they should and shouldn't do to help their children. The chaos and consequences of children using substances only multiplies a mom's obsessive and intrusive thoughts. These excessive interruptions deplete our energy and divert our focus.

You're Giving Away an Asset Called Attention

Getting hacked comes with a price more costly than dollars and cents. By adopting the role of worrier or fixer rather than creator and peacemaker, moms fail to embody their divine destiny. We get doubly hacked—first by one or more of those hacks I mentioned above that want our attention, then by our children's illness.

Let me clarify: Your children are worth your love and your fight. But if you find yourself constantly diverted, running in circles, and continually putting out fires, you'll miss opportunities to be guided in a more positive direction to do the right thing, and you won't be able to leave the legacy you always wanted. To stop the addiction stigma and find evidence-based recovery programs for your children, you must stay focused. There's a right way to win the attention war and a wrong way.

And there is a better way.

Through this multidisciplinary exploration of neurobiology, productivity, art, science, technology, athletics, military, and business, you'll soon discover the unmistakable elixir behind how to stay focused. This secret weapon is now available to aspiring mom super-achievers everywhere.

Ideas can change the world, but when moms get hacked and can't implement their ideas on how to change this addiction epidemic, no one wins. The thirty-day process in *Unhackable Moms of Addicted Loved Ones* will help you close the gap between havoc and hope. Once you find hope, you can start pursuing your dream and creating your legacy.

Abracadabra

Do you remember learning magic tricks as a child? You waved an imaginary wand over a hat or a towel, said, "Abracadabra," and pretended something instantly appeared. It was like saying, "Look at what I can do."

Abracadabra is made up of three Hebrew words: father, son, spirit. It means "I create as I speak." And it's literally translated, "It came to pass as it was spoken."

Linguists label it the most universally adopted word pronounced in other languages without need for translation.

Even as children, we loved magic tricks because the dreams in our hearts appeared just by speaking them.

Today, moms whose children suffer from an SUD wish they could speak the words, "Heal my child," and it would be done.

Unfortunately, healing never happens that way.

Isn't It Time for a New Story?

When our children were little, we read them bedtime stories. Sometimes the stories inspired them to think about a career. They'd say, "When I grow up, I want to be a policeman, or a pilot, or a teacher." In our daydreams, we saw them working in specific professions.

Once they started struggling with an SUD, they lost their jobs, cars, relationships, and everything they once owned. We grieved for the loss of dreams we had for them. But many of us never talked to anyone about our grief. We hid in shame.

Today, we tell story-lies to help us process our place in this world. We spin thousands of micro-stories every day. We say things like

- I am the cause of my child's problems.
- I can fix my child's SUD.
- I was a terrible mother.
- I've never been good at anything.
- No one values my opinion.
- I should have taken my child to the doctor sooner.

- I never should have taken that job.
- I should have divorced his father sooner.

These stories hold us back. They create prison bars around the possibilities. When we think about becoming *Unhackable Moms of Addicted Loved Ones*, it's easy to sabotage ourselves before we start. If we're not careful, we'll bring an old story along with us. We'll say things like . . .

- I'll never implement an idea because . . .
- I always get distracted because . . .
- I've never been very smart because . . .
- I can't follow through with what I want because . . .
- I don't have any ideas or dreams because . . .
- Even if I had a dream, I wouldn't be able to focus because. . .

The story we tell ourselves today often shapes our reality later. I've seen thousands of posts in our forum from moms who want their addicted loved one to seek recovery, yet they aren't seeking recovery for themselves. They often use one of these stories.

> Where your energy goes,
> your focus flows.
> **—Kary Oberbrunner**

Moms say we want our addicted loved ones to be more productive and focused on their recovery, yet we aren't seeking the same for ourselves.

If someone calls us out on how we're spending our time, we get defensive. We say, "You don't understand . . . ." We spend exorbitant amounts of time and energy trying to convince ourselves we don't need recovery; our child's addiction is not our problem. Yet we waste energy and emotion worrying instead of living our lives or building our legacy.

Essentially, we stack the deck in the enemy's favor by directing our creative power toward unproductive action.

It's important to note, we can't get off the havoc cycle without a support team. Rather than making unsuccessful attempts to drop the bad habits, we must replace them with good ones and surround ourselves with a team of moms who understand. This yields productive action.

We'll close this first day with a simple yet powerful exercise that will give you the ability to create a new story.

The Good News

You can become unhackable. Here are four of the most common benefits you can find if you apply this thirty-day *Unhackable* model:

- **Productivity:** Unhackable Moms are more productive. Without even realizing it, you will be able to let go of your obsessive thoughts and complete more tasks.

- **Fulfillment**: Unhackable Moms are more fulfilled. For the first time in a long time, you will feel more fully alive and filled with purpose to achieve what you want.

- **Focus**: Unhackable Moms are more focused. The daily method of taking little steps will allow you to gain clarity so interruptions can't control you.

- **Margin:** Unhackable Moms experience more margin. Margin is the amount of energy we hold in reserve for unanticipated situations. You will learn what to let go of and what to keep in your life so you can stay anchored to your God-given purpose and goal.

Up Until Now

Moms feel focusing on themselves makes them appear selfish. They wonder, "How can I think of anything except my sick child? Compassionate moms don't ignore their children for the sake of their own career or dreams."

When we focus on controlling others, however, we never win. We cannot control what our adult children do or don't do. Children do what children see—no matter their age. If we take charge of our own recovery and create a story for our future, others will notice. When moms recover, we become hope builders for our children.

Three powerful words make all the difference: *up until now.* If you begin using these words to write your future story, you will feel the power of planning a more desirable dream.

Let me show you what I mean. These are some of the examples that moms in the All-Mighty Mom Tribe shared:

Up until now . . . I haven't made myself a priority.

Up until now . . . I've allowed my thoughts to distract me from doing what I wanted.

Up until now . . . I've lost sleep and finances because of my addicted loved one.

Up until now . . . I've lost friends and family because of my child's problem.

Up until now . . . I've tried to control my child's choices.

Up until now . . . I've buffered the consequences of my addicted loved one's choices.

Up until now . . . I've assumed responsibility for my addicted loved one's choices, even though they weren't my fault.

Up until now . . . I quit before achieving my goals.

Up until now . . . I've let my addicted loved one hack my dreams.

Up until now . . . I didn't understand the consequences of my actions. I thought when my son went to detox, he would be done with active drug use.

Up until now . . . I paid my son's bills, which means I inadvertently bought his drugs.

Up until now . . . I haven't been able to sleep or stop obsessing about my addicted son. I couldn't stop thinking about the timeline for his recovery and thought it would happen quickly.

Up until now . . . The only person who mattered to me was my addicted son. I think of him first thing when I awake and throughout the day.

Up until now . . . All I thought about were ways to fix my son's problems.

Up until now . . . I was obsessed with finding a cure.

Up until now . . . I didn't believe my son had a drug problem.

Up until now . . . I haven't let God do His work.

Up until now . . . My whole life revolved around my addicted son.

These three words, *up until now*, will allow you to change your story rather than regurgitate the old one that subconsciously plays in your head. In a way, this phrase is a weapon to ward off the self-sabotaging thinking that's hacked you in the past and a way to deflect the enemy.

Up until now gives you permission to write a new story. Think of it as your first act of co-creation, a legitimate effort to return to your childhood. You'll sink your teeth into a simpler version of life once again. In this new world, you will . . .

- Create and implement an effective recovery plan for yourself.
- Engineer your attention and invest in the things you can control besides your addicted loved one's illness.

- Find and utilize the resources needed to pursue your child's recovery options so when he or she is ready, they can move toward building their dream.

- Exponentially increase your impact upon your addicted loved one and the world.

- Organize your life around flow—where you feel and perform your best.

Joy comes from the journey of working toward a dream and achieving it. That's what I want for you. To help you accomplish that, at the end of each day in this thirty-day plan, I'm going to challenge you with a clear action step.

CLOSE YOUR GAP—DAY 1: WRITE YOUR STORY

Today, I encourage you to write your story. By doing this, you give yourself permission to create a new future. Take this action to start closing the gap between havoc and hope. You'll discover how to become an Unhackable Mom of an Addict. Abracadabra is closer than you think.

In the past, what story have you told yourself to explain why you didn't achieve your goals? List as many micro-stories as possible.

Here are a few examples from moms in the Tribe:

- I didn't have the resources I needed.
- I didn't have people who supported me.
- I didn't have the necessary experience.
- My addicted child took all my time.

1. Does this past story serve your future dream?
2. Go back to your micro-stories and change the beginning. Insert the words "Up until now."

Your micro-stories should now look like this:

- *Up until now*, I didn't have the resources I needed.
- *Up until now*, I didn't have people who supported me.
- *Up until now*, I didn't have the necessary experience.
- *Up until now*, my addicted child took all my time.

Now, write your new story. Rather than focusing on what you don't have, write what you want instead. Don't write in the future tense—*I will have,* or *I will be*. Instead, write in the present tense—*I have* or *I am*.

Notes from the All-Mighty Mom Tribe

Dawn

I'm about to retire at age seventy. I can't even begin to think about doing anything for others or myself because I am concentrating on my son who struggles with alcoholism. I seriously have no aspirations. None. Retirement should be a reward of sorts.

I don't want to be miserable anymore, but up until now, I haven't done anything about searching for what I want.

***

Brooke

I had the opportunity to finish my master's degree in social work at the University of Tennessee, all expenses paid.

I prepared Micah, my twenty-seven-year-old addicted son: "I will be unavailable every Thursday for the next two years. You will need to make sure you have gas in your car, clothing for work, and everything you need, at least on Thursdays." I reminded him of this every day for a month.

On the first day of classes, Micah ran out of gas at 7:00 a.m. on his way to work. I told him I could bring $5 in gas and put it in his car, but I had class in an hour and could not answer my phone again that day.

Exactly one hour later, he ran out of gas again. He said he had to drive to a work site and didn't have money for more gas.

Because I was in class and did not answer my phone, he left more than sixty-seven messages.

When I finally called back at 3:00 p.m., Micah cursed me because he lost his job.

Every Thursday was filled with the same type of events.

After a semester, I quit the MSSW program because it was too much to work, go to college, and raise a twenty-seven-year-old child.

Up until now . . . my obsessive and unreasonable thoughts about Micah dominated every situation I encountered.

Up until now . . . I haven't taken the steps to change my behavior so I can fulfill my dreams whether Micah is choosing good health or not.

Up until now . . . I haven't chosen to live a different way by making my life and job a priority.

***

Sandy

Up until now . . . I did not commit to change.

Up until now . . . I did not think about what I wanted to accomplish.

Up until now . . . I did not have a plan for the day.

Up until now . . . I wasted too much time on my iPad.

I have time and know how to plan for what I want to accomplish each day. I know how to structure my time to accomplish my goals and can do that each day. I will give myself permission to rest and relax as part of this process.

***

Lily

Up until now . . . we haven't set boundaries because we were putting out fires as they happened—cancelling debit and credit cards, hiding cash, and not feeling comfortable leaving him alone in our home.

Up until now . . . we haven't felt safe from the actions of his substance use disorder.

DAY 2

Pick Your Boon

Your pain can lead to your most treasured triumph.
—Michelle Weidenbenner

You are the hero in your story. Maybe you're like Katniss Everdeen in *The Hunger Games,* sacrificing your life for someone else, your addicted child. Or perhaps you're more like Luke Skywalker in *Star Wars*, focused on transforming into a superhero to save the world. If you've never realized your hero status or considered living your story and rewriting the ending, I hope you do because it's fun and empowering.

As you write your story, you'll find there are three essential stages in every hero's journey.

The Departure

The story begins with departure. The hero ventures from her familiar world as she accepts the call to adventure. We enter this stage when something motivates us to leave our ordinary life behind and travel to a place we haven't been before. Inevitably, we approach a fork in the road. We must choose which path to travel, but once we start, there's no going back.

The Initiation

During the second stage, the hero learns to navigate the unfamiliar world. Perhaps this is where you are right now. As your child struggles with an SUD, you find yourself in uncharted territory. You lack experience, and you're not sure what to do, but there's no turning back because you accepted this call. In this present reality, you will hurdle obstacles, trudge through thunderstorms, and slip on icy terrain.

The Return

As you enter this third stage, I want to come alongside you as your guide. It will be my pleasure to help you return to your familiar world. This stage offers transformation. We can recapture the person God created you to be, a person made stronger and wiser by navigating the difficulties encountered along your journey. In the end, you'll find your most valued gift.

Your new world will be different from when you accepted the call to adventure because you've grown more resilient and learned new skills from traveling through the ups and downs. When you return to your familiar world, your addicted loved one may still be in the throes of addiction. You can't control that, but you will have the skills necessary to love him through his problem and will have started to overcome your attachment to it.

You have received this call to adventure; otherwise, you wouldn't be reading this book. You want help along your journey, and you've come to the right place. You will face a road of trials, but in the end, you will receive a great gift, your Boon.

By taking this thirty-day journey, you have accepted the call. You're ready for positive change. Many moms refuse the call. They don't want to change. They're afraid to try something new or travel to unknown places. Without knowing what you will find at the end of your transformation, you have committed to this journey because you and your child are worth the fight. Like many moms with addicted children, your health suffers, and nothing has worked, so you're willing to try something new. Your dedication to finding peace and learning how to change your present circumstances drives you.

You don't know what gift awaits you, but creating a Boon will help motivate you to recover and change.

What Is a Boon?

A Boon is a gift the hero receives as a reward for achieving her goals. Different heroes have different rewards, but all boons share a common characteristic: the boon gift has great value. Sometimes the Boon is used to improve the world.

A Boon is your deepest desire, your greatest ache, your deepest longing. Achieving your Boon holds intrinsic and extrinsic value. The intrinsic value might be the self-esteem you build as you accomplish the goal or the satisfaction of helping others. The extrinsic value for achieving your Boon might be seeing the physical results.

My Boon for this stage of my journey, for example, is to publish this book. My external reward is to see it come to life and hold the finished product in my hand. The internal reward is knowing my creation will help someone on a similar journey.

Dorothy, in *The Wizard of Oz,* wanted to return home. Her external Boon was to find her way back and be surrounded by her family again. Her internal reward came from the satisfaction of helping the scarecrow, tin man, and lion receive their gifts.

You might not know exactly what your Boon is in this moment, but the gift doesn't have to be clear. No one sees her

Boon perfectly in the beginning. Consider characters from movies or books; they set out in the ordinary world, unaware of how things are going to change. They seldom know what they want at the beginning of their story. But like it does with them, clarity will come to you as you act.

Picture yourself in a fog. With each step forward, the fog thins. It's not until you've walked a while through the fog that you will see your Boon. Many moms don't take those first steps. They get stuck, paralyzed in fear. You are different. I'm proud of you for taking the first step to walk through the fog.

Also, it's important to note, you will probably have more than one Boon in your lifetime. I've published nine books, each one a different Boon. For simplicity's sake through this thirty-day process, we're going to stick to one Boon.

You might use your Boon to improve the world, write a book, learn how to speak your story, work in a homeless shelter, or go back to college. Each person's Boon is unique, but having one will help you navigate the difficult life of coping with an addicted child. When we focus on our goal, there isn't time or energy to focus on our ALO.

How One Mom Achieved Her Boon

Courtney, a mom like you, became paralyzed with fear of losing her addicted loved one. She chose to embark on a journey and found her Boon along the way. Today, her efforts are exponentially multiplying. She is changing lives.

While Courtney's son lived in active addiction, she woke with her school-aged daughters, made their breakfast and lunch, drove them to school, and then went back to bed until it was time to pick them up.

She felt guilty for the trauma her son had experienced in his first seven years of his life while she was married to his father.

Her current husband, the father of their three daughters, climbed into bed beside her and said, "You need a shower."

"Really?"

"You stink."

It was her wake-up call. She vowed to shower once every three days and cook twice a week. It wasn't much, but it was a start.

On one of her most difficult days, she received a call from a respected man in her community, someone who knew her well and helped get people into recovery. "We need someone in the community to help educate parents. I can't help the families plus the addicts, but parents need education. You'd be great at leading them. Why don't you take this SMART Recovery class so you can facilitate a program to help out?"

Still not fully awake, Courtney mumbled that she would check it out. Then she hung up and went back to sleep.

Two weeks later, Mickey called her again. "Did you look into getting certified for the SMART Recovery program?"

"Uh, well. I forgot the name of the program. I didn't write down the information. Can you give it to me again?"

Courtney didn't know it at the time, but she was being called to do more, to turn her pain into purpose. She enrolled in the course. It became the baby step that got her out of bed and propelled her toward her Boon.

I met Courtney Jenkins in a small conference room at a coffee shop in an addiction support meeting, a place to share my frustrations about having a son in addiction. It was my first visit. She was facilitating.

When the sitting sheriff received a grant to start a Jail Chemical Addiction Program (JCAP), Courtney wanted to be involved. Facilitating the women's Self-Management and Recovery Training (SMART) groups allowed her to do that.

Her son's struggle with addiction motivated her to do more in the jail. She'd seen too many get out and use again, proving their stay was ineffective.

She volunteered for months before a new sheriff took office and asked her to step in, coordinate, and build the JCAP program into what she thought it could and should be. Since she took the reins, people in the community have rallied to take part in the transformation of the select group of men and women who go through this four-month program.

Courtney didn't plan to take over the SMART program when she started volunteering at the jail. She had to walk through the fog one step at a time. Along the way she faced trials. In the beginning, none of the jail staff approved of her. Though strictly a volunteer position, they thought she made more money than them. It took months and months of showing up and pouring into these broken souls for her to gain their respect. She didn't let their unacceptance stop her.

Her initial Boon was to encourage parents of addicted children by leading SMART recovery, but she also saw another need: educating the women prisoners. Courtney's Boon didn't have anything to do with her son's recovery or if he was still using because she couldn't control her son's behavior. All she could do for herself was move forward on her journey to help others. Seeing what her son was going through helped her understand persons with criminal backgrounds and SUDs.

Working with the women at the jail led to more opportunities. Her Boon expanded to the men in the jail. Today she has served more than sixty-five incarcerated people. By getting others in her community involved in her work, she has helped to lessen the stigma of incarceration and reduce recidivism.

Courtney didn't see all the great things that would happen when she first set out to encourage others who were struggling, but by taking the first step, she was able to comfort other parents and then see incarcerated people beat their SUD and become productive citizens. They gave her hope for her son and helped her regain control of her life and contribute to others in meaningful ways.

It all started with an encouraging phone call from someone who believed in Courtney. That belief nourished a withered seed of hope and brought back to life the desire to do something more. When she took the first step, she didn't know where the path would ultimately lead. It wasn't until months after she began to facilitate the SMART program that she understood the full rewards of her involvement. An even bigger Boon may still await her down the road, but she can't see it yet.

Like Courtney, we can put our pain to great use, too, if we look outside the narrow window of our own child's problem. What makes you laugh? What makes you angry? What makes you cry? What is one little thing you can do today to change the addiction landscape in your community?

I want to help you walk through your fog and come out in the clearing with a better idea of what your Boon will be, even if it's a tiny step. I am confident God has given you the ability to recover so you can use your gifts to build up the Kingdom.

Below you'll find stories of moms who have a dream for their recovery. They visualize where they want to be at the end of this journey.

CLOSE YOUR GAP DAY 2: PICK YOUR BOON

1. What is your deepest desire, your greatest ache, your truest longing? Journal everything that comes to mind. Don't edit and don't focus on being correct.

2. If you still need help picking your Boon, talk to your friends and family members who know you well. Ask them what gifts they see in you. Do a mental autopsy. What makes you angry? What breaks your heart? What

is it that keeps you hopeless? What's a big problem that you want to solve? Make a list.

3. Visualize what your life will look like after you've achieved your Boon. Create positive images of a new future. Let go of all attachment to a specific outcome.

4. Answer these questions openly and honestly, with the first thing that pops into your mind.

5. If you're ambitious, visit HavocToHope.com to find questions that will help you pick your Boon.

Note: Your Boon can't be for your child to choose recovery. Yes, we all want that, but we can't control their lives. We must focus on what we can do despite their illness. Your Boon is about you and what you want to create, accomplish, or achieve.

If your Boon isn't clear yet, don't worry. There will be time to fine-tune it later. As you will see in the Boon samples below, some of our tribe's Boons are unclear too. This is a new concept for most of us and doesn't jump out immediately.

Notes from the All-Mighty Mom Tribe

As you read the excerpts below, notice that some moms have difficulty identifying their Boon. This is normal. The concept is new to many of us. Don't be discouraged if you lack clarity in this section. Journal your thoughts and keep going. Clarity will come with action.

Sally

I plan to minister to mothers of addicted children. I want to help them find scriptures to pray and teach them the promises of God that are all yes and amen. I will demonstrate ways to believe and invest time in themselves so they can be the women of faith and leaders God called them to be. Then they will be empowered to look outside themselves and begin ministering to others.

***

Brooke

I sit on the board of directors for a nonprofit formed to build tiny home villages for those coming out of rehabilitation or jail. We received two apartment buildings as gifts recently and are in the process of getting a sprinkler system installed to meet state codes so these can be used as transitional housing. We are also in the planning stages of building a second village on a piece of property of another nonprofit, Century Harvest Farms. They assist with job training and employment.

Helping people in the same situation as my son has been a very interesting experience. Many times, I provided my son with housing. I paid for apartments, bought a trailer and a house. Still, he could not remain sober or maintain even the smallest of expectations, so I couldn't help him. When he was sober, he wanted to help those without homes, and I've always had that desire also. When the opportunity came to help our community with an affordable housing crisis, I decided to help. Here's our organization: pivottn.org.

***

Lori

I would love to take my family's land and grow seasonal flowers and produce to sell in a small roadside store. I would love to have the opportunity to employ those who suffer from addiction and need help getting on their feet.

***

Sandy

I will continue to be active in Moms Letting Go Without Giving Up, Moms of Addicted Loved Ones, and the lives of friends and acquaintances who struggle emotionally. I will pray for specific needs and respond with encouraging thoughts and words. I will listen without judgment and do all I can to help connect other moms with needed resources.

***

Lucretia

My Boon is to find peace at a cabin by the beach reflecting with God, walking in the sand, and chilling. But my Boon is also to speak passionately to other moms so I can ignite them to be the best they can be and live an abundant life.

DAY 3

Identify Your Enemy

Mastering others is strength; mastering oneself is true power.
—Lao Tsu

Our granddaughters (eleven and sixteen years old) participate in a water ski show team. Every summer, the girls
practice three times a week and perform in two shows a week.
They love their ski family and enjoy spending their summers
with them on the water, not only because it's challenging but
also because working with four-year-olds to fifty-year-olds
brings many different perspectives to their lives.

They perform many stunts, including building human
pyramids and strap doubles. Skiers build pyramids by standing
on the shoulders of other performers who stand on the shoulders of the base skiers. In strap double performances, a base
skier (male) attaches the ski rope to a belt around his waist.
A female skier rides on his shoulders, ready to be lifted in the
air. She performs handstands, death drops, and torch flips. In
between, they smile at the audience in their glittery costumes,
and she points her toes. When they compete, they're scored

on how straight their lines are and how well they interact with the audience.

At practice one evening, a young skier wanted to take off from the dock with a girl on his shoulders. No girl would go. Nine-year-old Addie felt sorry for him, so she agreed to join him—not once, but three times. Each time, she fell because he wasn't strong enough to hold her up. And each time, she hit a ski. Later that night, she complained about her beat-up shins. She told us she didn't want to go, but no one else would, so she thought she should.

"What could you have done?" I asked Addie.

She shrugged. "I don't know."

"You had a choice. You could have said no."

She looked away.

"What would have happened if you'd said no?" I asked.

She shrugged again.

"If you hadn't gone off the dock on his shoulders, you wouldn't have fallen and hurt yourself."

"But nobody would go with him, and I felt sorry for him," she said.

"So, to make him feel better, you hurt yourself, even though you knew after the first time he couldn't hold you?"

She nodded.

This event allowed me to illustrate the importance of saying no and how powerful our choices are. Addie wanted people to like her. She's sensitive and intuitive about how other people feel. She's too young to recognize this as a gift—one that many other people don't have—but without boundaries, the gift can quickly become a curse.

Addie's not the only people-pleaser. Many moms want to be liked by their children and others too. No one taught them how to set boundaries; therefore, they didn't learn an important leadership skill—how to lead themselves and guard their self-care.

"Who is the most important person you'll ever lead?" I asked Addie.

She paused for a minute. "My children?"

"They will be important someday, for sure, but there's someone even more important."

"Who?" she asked.

"You are the most important person you'll ever lead. Who is responsible for those spills you took on the water?"

"He was."

"Think again," I said.

"Okay, Mimi. I get it. It was me. I should have said no."

I don't know if she learned anything that day, but when I asked her if she wanted to practice saying no with me, she said, "No!"

Moms Worry Best

Anxiety disorders affect forty million adults, according to the Anxiety and Depression Association of America (ADAA). In other words, they affect about 18 percent of the U.S. population, which makes them the most common type of mental illness in the United States.[7]

The study doesn't say how many of these adults are moms of addicted loved ones, but I know that most moms with these kids worry.

How do I know?

When moms of addicted loved ones ask to join my private Facebook group, Moms Letting Go, they must answer three questions before they're approved. One is this: What is your greatest fear? Ninety-eight percent of them answer that they fear their child will die of an overdose. The other 2 percent worry their children will end up in prison or jail and/or destroy the rest of their lives.

Every day, moms worry about something that might never happen. Our imaginations take over because we know the faceless enemy called addiction is real and ugly. The news reports overdose deaths driven by synthetic opioids like fentanyl spiked after the start of the pandemic. According to the National Center for Health Statistics, more than 270 people die every day of overdoses, and fentanyl is a killer that is starting to be found in almost every substance.[8]

Even those moms who don't read the news know the dangers of fentanyl because we see our children's addicted friends dying. The stakes are high, and so are our worries.

One of my favorite Bible verses is Matthew 6:27 (NIV): "Can any one of you by worrying add a single hour to your life?" Though we know worry doesn't add value to our lives or our children's lives, it doesn't mean we know how to stop. Yet. (We will learn more tips on how to stop obsessive thoughts another day.)

Who Is Your Enemy?

You have an enemy. He's been working to sabotage you your entire life. Whenever you dream and set out to achieve it, this spiritual enemy brings the burden of your addicted loved one's SUD down on you. The pressure weighs heavy; it leaves you feeling depressed and unable to stand tall, let alone tackle your dream. You lack the energy to do anything, and if you find time to do something joyful, exhaustion steals your creativity and drive. Amid the havoc, you get lost and so does your hope.

We often feel like we scored the lead role in a thriller. But our reality is more like a nightmare. Our thoughts, dreams, and hope get hacked.

We self-sabotage by allowing the chaos to rule. We become addicted to the addiction cycle and blame our lack of focus on someone else. Our enemy knows if he can convince us someone else caused our misery, he wins.

Addiction is a spiritual battle, and the enemy thrives on hacking us. He works to keep our ALOs out of recovery because he sees how it affects us. When we focus on our own recovery and recognize the spiritual enemy against us, overcoming the obstacles becomes achievable.

Now for the Good News

Your adversary can be defeated! Yes, it takes introspection and truth-telling, but we are mighty women. We can take the medicine.

Do you remember your Boon from Day Two? It may have been difficult to put into words, but hopefully you wrote something down. To recap, your Boon is your deepest desire, your greatest ache, or your truest longing—something that's been inside you longer than the desire, ache, and longing for your child.

Look at the chart below.

On the left side, list your current situation or present experience. This is your old story that held you back on Day One. When you wrote, "Up until now," what were those limitations you cited?

On the right side, list a few thoughts about your Boon and your future expectations. Don't worry if it's vague. Aim for imperfect action. Remember, clarity only comes with action.

PRESENT EXPERIENCE	HACKED	FUTURE EXPECTATIONS

Between your future expectations and your present experience lies a list of hackers—people or circumstances keeping you from joy. Without deep thinking, quickly list all the people and things in your way under the HACKED column. What or who makes it difficult for you to live a joy-filled, Boon-achieving life?

Once you've completed the center column, review your list. Do you see any patterns in these hacks? Write your observations below:

_____

_____

_____

_____

Did certain names keep showing up? What about specific actions or circumstances?

When my younger self did this exercise, my husband's job, my children, and lack of available time topped the list of things holding me back. For years, I used this list as an excuse to not work toward my dream. I complained. I tried to write during my spare time and got side-tracked by a sick kid or one of their sports functions. I blamed some of it on my husband being out of town for work. There was never any time left for me between paying the bills, managing the kids, and running the household.

Today I Know Differently

Now I know differently. Maybe it's my age; I'm older and wiser. Or maybe I learned from listening to my son's and daughter-in-law's excuses when they lived in the throes of addiction. They never took responsibility for their choices. I used to call it blame-itis. (You won't find that word in the dictionary, but I used it whenever they blamed someone or something else for their havoc.)

> I have learned over the years that when one's mind is made up, this diminishes fear; knowing what must be done does away with fear.
> **—Rosa Parks**

Wherever I go, there I am. If we can't lead ourselves well, it's easy to blame others when we fail. Addie wanted to blame her friend when he kept dropping her in the water. Blaming others, making excuses, and living in denial will not solve the problem, but any one of those will prolong the pain. Until we own our role in the story and our ability to change the outcome, we will remain stuck.

Victim or a Victor?

How do you view yourself?

When we view ourselves as powerless victims, our lives become reactive. We lie in a BED of blame, excuses, and denial.

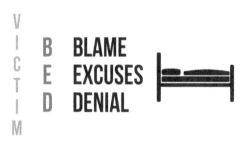

Consider your addicted child. List his excuses: Why he doesn't have money. Why he lost his job or his phone. Pay attention to whom he blames and the explanations he gives.

If we help our children live this lie—life is happening *to* them, and they have no role in their story—we help prolong their pain. Likewise, when we use our ALO as an excuse for our lack of joy or hope, we prolong our pain.

We become our own worst enemy.

Yes, other people and circumstances can hack us, but how we choose to respond to those flat tires, contagious viruses, deaths in the family, and more makes a difference. We have a choice. We can remain a victim, allowing things beyond our control to keep us from a fulfilling life, or develop a victor mindset and become proactive about our future.

While a victim lies in BED, a victor moves forward with OAR: ownership, accountability, and responsibility. You can become a victor. When moms become victors, they create hope for their children. Children imitate what they see. When they see us taking OAR, they will learn from the best.

```
V
I        O    Ownership
C        A    Accountability
T        R    Responsibility
O
R
```

Victors take ownership of their life. They desire account-ability, and rather than focusing on the wrongs others have committed, they recognize their responsibility in their lack of joy and hope. Victors make difficult choices, set healthy boundaries, and advocate for themselves. When we choose to live as a victor, we learn to respond to hackers instead of reacting.

Knee-jerk reactions add to the pain; we say things we don't mean and make rash decisions that alleviate the immediate crisis but make the long-term situation worse. On the other hand, thought-out responses bring words of truth, sometimes hard to hear, but with the potential to bring healing. They convey boundaries and allow you to take ownership and responsibility of your life.

CLOSE YOUR GAP DAY 3: IDENTIFY YOUR ENEMY

Who is hacking you? Who is your enemy? None of us wants to get hacked, but when it happens, it's our responsibility to handle the hack with OAR.

Admitting we hack ourselves is a step toward healing. When we recognize we get in our own way and we're our own worst enemy, we find hope and can claim our All-Mighty Mom status.

Each hero chooses which fork in the road she will take on her journey. Luke Skywalker had to choose between answering Leia's plea or remaining a farm boy. Katniss Everdeen decided to participate in the Hunger Games rather than watch her sister and the rest of her community die.

We can choose the path that allows our ALOs to continue to hack our lives, or we can choose to rise above and embrace the responsibility to change. Do you want to . . .

- become a proactive victor?
- own your pattern for getting hacked?
- become accountable for your hacking problem?
- embrace your responsibility for the need to change?

You have a second option. You can stay in your comfort zone and deny your role as the enemy, but you'll stay stuck too. If you decide not to do anything, you will . . .

- remain a reactive victim,
- continue blaming your addicted loved one for your life,
- keep making excuses for why you're getting hacked, and
- live in denial about the fact that you have become your own enemy.

Change requires commitment. Your choice will make you or break you. Are you ready?

Write your commitment below and date it.

I, _____, hereby declare, as of this date, _____, I will embrace my OARs and no longer allow my BED to get in the way of reaching my dreams, goals, or Boon.

_____   _____
Signature   Witness or Accountability Partner

Notes from the All-Mighty Mom Tribe

Lori

I was the enemy, trying to control everything. I didn't want to see what was right before my eyes. Making excuses, I wanted to believe my son. Surely, he wouldn't lie and steal from me! Ha! He lied right to my face. Then came the days when I could not ignore the signs anymore. I had to act—either sink or swim. Living as a victim is not living; it's existing. I knew God wanted me to experience abundant life. I began to realize my plan and God's plan had to be on the same page. I had serious health concerns, and as I lost control, I lost my family too.

***

Brooke

I have been the enemy in my story. I have been so addicted to my son, attempting to "make" him recover, that I lost my way.

It all stemmed from my desire to be a good, supportive parent. I didn't have this type of role model; I wanted to be different for my children. I longed for a close and loving relationship. When Micah's addiction took over, I chased after him in unbelievable situations, trying to force him toward recovery.

I hacked myself. My family is in shambles, my career stalled, I'm addicted to my son, and I feel responsible for all the failure.

On this day, I will begin a slow process of change. I will begin finding the things that make me feel alive, and I will start doing them more often. I will let myself feel love from my husband, my friends, and my dogs. I will move forward in a more purposeful and productive way.

***

Darra

I know I am the enemy because I am the one with anger and resentment. I have invested in a counselor to talk about this spiritual battle. This past week we talked about how the greatest enemies are the ones in my own home. I can't control them, but I must love, feed, and pray for my enemies.

***

Lily

I've been hacked because, in addition to my son's substance abuse issues and the damage those created, I'm facing major health problems with some of my other close family members. My retirement plans always included travel, and now those plans are in limbo. I want it all to go away. But this is my life now. I'm owning that. I am accountable and responsible for my life decisions and how I respond to these major issues in my life. I'm seeking therapy to cope with these situations and have been diagnosed with adjustment disorder with anxiety, which means I'm having trouble adjusting to being hacked. I turn to God for help with all this, and ultimately I know I will be fine. He will help me navigate these challenges. It's just a lot to handle all at once.

DAY 4

Seize Your Saboteur

*The enemy doesn't stand a chance
when the victim decides to survive.*
—Rae Smith

A re you in danger of someone hacking your bank account? I hope not, but it happens; therefore, banks now demand we set safety precautions. Sometimes it takes four different passcodes to get into our accounts. It's annoying but necessary.

Human hacking might be worse because we don't see our part. Yes, we often become the saboteurs. Self-sabotage happens when we let our behaviors and thought patterns prevent us from being the person God created us to be.

As moms of addicted loved ones, we get defensive, feeling like our child's problems stem from our poor parenting. We stay connected to our phones, even when we sleep, every second waiting for our child to text so we know he's okay. Some moms work two jobs to help pay their addicted child's rent and child support because they feel guilty. We cancel plans with friends and family and ignore our spouses and other children because we're hyper-focused on our sick child.

I asked moms in our private Facebook group, Moms Letting Go, "Why do we over-apologize?" Here are a few of their answers:

- I'm embarrassed that my son chooses heroin over everything else.
- I'm embarrassed for his children.
- I don't want to be judged.
- I feel guilty for his poor choices because he blames me for putting him on Ritalin for ADHD when he was a child.
- I would never do what he does, so it feels bad when I know others are watching him.
- I think I failed as a mother.

Maybe you have felt like some of these mothers.

Catching your negative thoughts is an important step to changing. Awareness must come before we can change.

In the book, *Changing for Good*, Prochaska and DiClemente describe six stages of change. Understanding these stages helps us have realistic expectations for our children's recovery as well as our own ability to change. Read these stages with your loved one in mind, but go back and read them with your own recovery or change in mind.

The Stages of Change[9]

Stage 1: Precontemplation—Not ready to change. The person might not recognize the consequences of their actions. Some of our loved ones are court-ordered into treatment. They aren't changing their behavior because it's their choice but because they're pressured into treatment.

Stage 2: Contemplation—Thinking about change. The person might acknowledge their problem but probably doesn't have the confidence to take a step forward into change.

Stage 3: Preparation—Ready to change. The person is willing to take a small step forward. Setting small, achievable goals is helpful in this stage.

Stage 4: Action—Moving toward change. This person has developed plans for change and is implementing them. Their actions show they're working toward their goals.

Stage 5: Maintenance—Practicing the change. This is when the person has adopted the change for at least six months. They're committed to change and have implemented coping strategies to avoid temptation.

Stage 6: Termination—The goal is to complete the change goal, but this stage is often called the relapse stage. It's when the person has lapsed back into old behaviors. They feel frustration, disappointment, or have feelings of failure. The key is to support your loved one and encourage him to recommit to his goals.

Relapses happen to moms too. When we bend our boundaries and do something we used to do, instead of staying committed to our new boundary, we often experience a similar frustration and disappointment. We hack our lives through our own relapse, especially if our loved one is still in active addiction, and we're making it easy for them to stay in active addiction.

I wish the final stage was the *Transformation* stage because it sounds more positive and better describes my goal for you and your children; however, relapses happen. (We prefer to use the word "reoccurrence" instead of relapse. See Appendix D for using the proper addiction terms.)

In the final stage, with divine help, a metamorphosis can happen. I want to help you transform your life so your child's addiction doesn't hack your dreams into stagnation. Just remember that if you get to stage six and relapse, find a support partner to talk to and get back into your committed program.

Do you know what stage you are in? What stage is your child in?

Each of us is in a different stage. Even though we'd like to rush our addicted children through all six stages, this isn't going to happen. Expecting quick change sets us up for disappointment and resentment. If, however, we allow them to face the consequences of using—without throwing them a safety net—they will experience the adverse effects of their addiction and be willing to talk about making changes.

In a similar way, I've heard moms of addicted loved ones share their difficulties in our free support group. Many continue to repeat their co-dependent actions; they stay stuck in the cycle, ambivalent to change. These moms say they want to be different, but when their child calls or experiences a hardship, they bend their boundaries and throw the safety net again.

These women are not bad mothers. I've been there too. There are so many moving parts when we love a person with an SUD. I didn't know which boundaries to change, and I couldn't understand how *not helping* was going to help him. We can't see clearly or make good decisions when we're staring into the droopy, bloodshot eyes of our children as they self-destruct in front of us.

If you're still in stage one, not willing to seize your saboteur and recognize you have a problem, close this book and save it until you reach stage two. The mom who doesn't think she has a problem can't be helped. I empathize. I once thought, *It's my son's problem. Not mine.* Yet I was the one who couldn't sleep or breathe.

If you're ready to do the work, keep reading.

The Hack Attack

Kary Oberbrunner calls the effects of human hacking the Hack Attack.[10] It's a sophisticated sequence that systematically strips away eight essential components and leaves victims, like you, vulnerable and exposed. See if you have suffered one of these attacks.

You feel a loss of . . .

- control
- clarity
- competence
- confidence

- insight
- influence
- impact
- income

It's impossible to sort through the havoc in our lives and find hope when we've lost so much. The Hack Attack sounds something like this:

- I can't control what my addicted child says or does, nor can I control my obsessive thoughts. (Loss of control)
- I'm not sure how to help. If I give him too much, I'm enabling. If I detach and show him tough love, then how will he know I love him, and where will he find hope? (Loss of clarity)

- I'm a terrible mother and incapable of doing anything right. (Loss of competence)
- I'm an imposter. (Loss of confidence)
- I have no vision for my future. (Loss of insight)
- I have no effect on my addicted child. My child doesn't listen to me and tells me I don't understand. (Loss of influence)
- I have no credibility. I don't understand what is happening to my child or the disease of addiction. (Loss of impact)
- I have no currency because I've spent so much on helping him and finding professional recovery options. (Loss of income)

These Hack Attacks start externally in the lives of every person our ALOs meet, but they quickly manifest internally.

Many of the declarations above shape your perception of yourself, affecting your perspective on everything that happens to you.

Many moms of addicted loved ones believe these lies:

First lie: This problem is my fault.
Second lie: My child is going to die.
Third lie: I can't stop worrying.
Fourth lie: If I help him by throwing a safety net, he'll appreciate me, quit using, and get better.

When you believe these lies, you're done. You become frozen in fear and stay stuck in the muck of despair and the continuous chaotic cycle.

Thank God, you have the power to stop the Hack Attack before it kills you and your addicted child. You can seize your saboteur, put your dukes up and your claws out, and create a counterattack.

You can reverse what's happening to you and move closer to unhackability.

Unhackable Moms Are Outliers

An outlier mom stands out from the crowd, noticed for the positive way she leads herself, for her confidence, insight, influence, and vision, and for the way she takes responsibility for her choices and embraces clarity. You can become this mom. That's why you picked up this book. You're the exception. You might not be a bold outlier yet, but you will be after these thirty days.

Once you seize the sabotaging behaviors and thought patterns that are holding you back, you will be on your way to balancing bold boundaries, creating calm compassion, and knowing how to leave a loving legacy.

Your family, friends, and addicted loved one will see you differently. They'll learn about addiction and how to care without falling to pieces. They'll notice the change in you and find hope for themselves. And you will be living your authentic self.

CLOSE YOUR GAP DAY 4: SEIZE YOUR SABOTEUR

It's time to close your gap between havoc and hope.

First Step: Verbalize these eight new declarations about your identity and your resources. A Hack Counterattack empowers you to say

- I am in charge of my life. (Control)
- I am not confused. I know what to do and say. (Clarity)

- I am a good and capable mother. (Competence)
- I am authentic. (Confidence)
- I have a vision for my future. (Insight)
- I positively influence my addicted loved one. (Influence)
- I have credibility. (Impact)
- I have currency. (Income)

Second Step: Write these statements in your journal and say them out loud during your devotional time. Or stick them on your refrigerator so others can see what you're working on, and you'll be able to see the words every day. Once you believe these statements, you'll feel empowered to embrace them.

You'll never outperform your self-image, and until you reset how you see yourself, you'll keep getting hacked.

Third Step: Add these new truths to your list of things to remember. You didn't cause your child's addiction. You can't control the disease or cure it.

- Every person is going to die, including your child, but it won't be your fault. We will pray it won't be from an overdose, but we can't control what happens.
- Worrying doesn't change anyone. It keeps us locked in a prison of fear.
- Allowing our adult children to face the consequences of their actions helps them move into recovery sooner.

Fourth Step: List some counterattack tools that will help you. What will you commit to? Here are some suggestions:

- Join an online support group
- Join a private Facebook group

- Hire a private recovery coach
- Attend local community meetings
- Talk to a recovering addict and learn what his/her mom and dad did to help them recover
- Gather a list of questions that will help you say no
- Listen to addiction podcasts
- Join a Bible study

Notes from the All-Mighty Mom Tribe

Lucretia

When my addicted son got his girlfriend pregnant, I knew the chaos had to stop. This was the second time he'd fathered a child. I didn't want to go through the difficulty again. My brain couldn't take it anymore. I had to seize what was hacking me, so I asked a few of my good friends to commit to praying for me and my family. My husband and I met with our pastor and prayed about our situation. I was completing a Bible study locally and enrolled in an online Bible study too. I started gathering information. I read books, researched Celebrate Recovery, called organizations and doctor friends. Online, I searched for addiction information that would help me move forward. I cried a lot and prayed a lot, and I didn't sleep well. I wanted to get comfortable in our county courthouse so I could see what other pending charges my son was facing. It was all coming to a head, but I had to let go and have faith. My strength was fading.

***

Teresa

Before I started my own recovery, I had enabled my son for years. I paid for things I shouldn't have, like cell phones, gas for his car, or for friends who drove him when his car got impounded. I funded his trip to the methadone clinic, as well as motels and groceries when he wasn't living with us, not to mention the deductible on a car he borrowed and wrecked. I gave him cash and drove him to buy meds on the street so he wouldn't be sick from withdrawals. I wired money to him several times after he had been kicked out of our house. So much money spent—usually without my husband knowing.

I gave up many hours of sick leave and vacation time, plus weekends "saving him" from difficult situations. I took him food, was there for him on court dates, and visited him in jail. I believed him when he said the methadone clinic set him up at a recovery facility ninety miles away. I took him to breakfast and told him how proud I was. But when we got to the rehab place, they knew nothing about him and had no room available.

Less than two months later, he was arrested for the first time for selling methadone.

My own recovery started after many years of co-dependent behavior. I finally realized all my "help" was not changing my son's behavior. I was at my wit's end and exhausted emotionally and physically. My marriage was on the brink of failure. I went to Celebrate Recovery at the advice of a friend and did the nine-month study program. That led to women's retreats and a Bible study group that has been my rock, along with God, of course! I started to learn about addiction. Then I found this online Tribe of Mighty Moms who really understand, teach, and support me in my ever-continuing journey to recover, even though my son still chooses not to be in recovery.

***

Brooke

Since I have seen the downside of living with addiction, I tried very hard to keep my son from going down the same road as other family members. Despite my best efforts, Micah became addicted to alcohol, and I became addicted to Micah, throwing every solution in the book at his issues. I tried everything to make him stop, to keep consequences from damaging him, and to prevent the rest of the family from suffering.

One night Micah came home so drunk he couldn't walk through the front door. He had driven himself home but fell on the front porch. I did not want my in-laws to see—I was newly married, and they lived next door—so I dragged his 200-pound body in the house and managed to get him on the couch. I put cold rags on his face and body, trying to revive him.

He laughed when he felt the cold water. His eyes danced back and forth. He seemed so happy in his fantasy world.

I finally realized the futility of my efforts and sat with his head in my lap. I cried and prayed.

A few hours later, Micah woke up and said, "Momma, what's wrong with you?"

I had cried until there were dark circles around my eyes and red splotches on my face. I told him I was sad about the state he was in.

"I was happy. Go to bed," he said.

At times, I realize I am the crazy one in the relationship because I am addicted to a grown child I cannot control. This time, I made a vow to stop letting someone else's actions control my life.

I have had many lessons to learn, and recovery has been like a slow peeling onion, one tiny layer at a time. I wish there were a switch I could flip and feel healed, but for me, the changes are very small and taking lots of time.

***

Lucretia

My resentment and bitterness were growing day by day as I continued to add to the long list of where my money was going. I thought I was helping; sure, he would wake up one day soon and get his life together. With a grandchild who must be cared for, I was willing to do just about anything to make that happen.

Finally, I had a "come to Jesus" meeting and realized we had spent thousands on him and his baby momma. Food, utilities, gas, car, insurance, day care, clothes, doctors, medicines, and yes, we even let them move back home. The realization helped me decide I needed to change my response to my son's requests. I couldn't continue to let him hack my finances.

Count Your Cost

Lost time is never found again.
—Benjamin Franklin

I sat in the pew that Sunday trying to hold back tears. A family I knew well sat to my right. Articulate, warm, and engaging, they spent a lot of time together. The parents dressed neatly, smiled, and held hands. Their high-school-aged children participated in Future Business Leaders Association, volunteered at the homeless shelter, and were in the honor society. I doubted their children experimented with alcohol or marijuana.

To the left and up a few pews, sat the fifth-grade teacher who predicted we'd have problems with Ryan, our son. One fall, I attended his parent-teacher conference alone. As usual, my husband had to travel for work. Once Ryan's teacher started, her comments spilled over with foaming anger, obviously frustrated with our son. Without my husband to defend me and our son, I felt attacked. I was doing the best I could but often felt judged as a poor parent.

Mom guilt starts early. We compare ourselves with other moms whose kids don't act out, talk back, experiment with substances, or have ADHD. We look at these moms and wonder what they do that we don't do. We compare and feel inferior.

That mom guilt kept me locked in a place that gobbled hours and years of my time. I read parenting books trying to figure out how to be a better mom. Self-limiting beliefs made me hesitant and inconsistent with behavior consequences. I confused my son by setting weak boundaries. I neglected my other children. I was mentally unavailable. Every waking hour, my thoughts steered to my son's chronic rebellion. At night, nightmares hacked my dreams. With each job, I felt like a failure. I couldn't juggle the home, kids, and my job, so I quit. Quitter became one of my new names.

That Sunday in church I could have focused on praying for my son, felt pride for who he was, and accepted God had a plan for him. Instead, I obsessed over figuring out my mistakes and finding different approaches. I wasn't aware of how much it was distracting me and costing my family.

I don't want you to make the same mistakes. Addiction tears apart marriages and family relationships. The havoc your children's addiction causes will hack you, too, if you don't find a recovery plan.

Moms are afraid of change, just like their addicted children.

One mom in our support group said, "I wish I could get back the time I spent trying to save my addicted children. I wish I had focused on the family that needed me home."

What if staying stuck guarantees your child won't recover? There are no assurances your efforts will change your child. When moms and dads throw a safety net, bail their children out of jail, or make excuses for their choices, it can prolong their addiction because the child doesn't have to take the consequences of his actions. Not until the pain of using is greater than the pleasure will a person be motivated to change.

Each time you try to protect your child, there is a cost. The energy you expend on your child prevents you from having the energy to create your legacy. Spinning in the chaos cycle leaves no energy for living your dream life, and constantly saving our children from the consequences of their actions leaves us empty.

Every day in the private Facebook group, moms ask for suggestions on how to help their children, but some never try anything new. These stuck moms post a similar question two weeks later, ignoring the advice they received earlier.

Fear of Change

Insanity is doing the same thing over and over again and expecting different results. If we want a new outcome, we must change our actions. Instead of worrying about the future and imagining negative outcomes, it's time to envision positive results from our actions.

Have you heard the new acronym FOMO? Many have it, but what if we could use fear of missing out to our benefit?

What if you could see what your life would look like if you hadn't gotten hacked by your child's addiction? Imagine life if you had spent your time, resources, and finances fulfilling your Boon. Let that picture create FOMO for your Boon.

Reach for this new acronym in your life: JOMO. Joy of missing out. It's when we choose to miss out on the drama in our lives so we find joy.

There's a cost associated with not achieving this new self. It's an expense, not only to you and your family but to the world. When we stay stuck, the enemy laughs because our contribution to society is minimized. He gets two hacks for the price of one—you and your addicted child.

Even if your Boon is to find peace so you can live in your sweet spot, it is a gift given to you and for you. It's entrusted to you. Once you're able to share your healed self, you will be able to lead others.

Fear of Commitment

I can't do this.

I can't think of myself when my child is suffering.

It's selfish to focus on my needs.

Who does this sound like? The excuses keep coming. It gets worse when our friends and family share their opinions.

Aren't you going to do anything to make them stop?

How can you leave your child homeless?

Your child is embarrassing the family.

Keep this hidden.

Bail him out of jail.

Call the newspaper and pay them to keep his photo out of the paper.

You need to let her live with you.

When we listen to our self-doubts and the uneducated advice from our friends and family, we get hacked. We stop self-progress and freeze in fear.

Fear Is Real

Refer to the Boon you identified on Day 2. What fear stops you from committing to your dreams? Be honest about what scares you.

What if you flipped your focus? Instead of thinking about what you'll gain if you pursue your Boon, think of what you'll lose. What will staying stuck cost you if you never detach from owning your adult children's problems? What will your family and society lose if you don't follow your dream to leave a legacy?

I keep a file of the positive comments moms have made about the steps I've taken to achieve my Boon—to empower one million moms of addicted loved ones into recovery by 2025. When I feel discouraged, I read them. They encourage me to keep going.

Doing so has brought me closer to God. I give Him the glory to keep my ego out. This mission is not about me. It's about focusing on God who reminds me why I have this Boon and where He is calling me.

Here are a few of those testimonials I keep in my file:

I went to the cardiologist today, and when I told him how much I sleep every day, I realized how much I've been trying to escape. I'm reading your book and reciting some of the lines repeatedly. Thank you for writing this book!

***

I appreciate you sharing your courage, vulnerability, and hope.

***

Thank you for the inspiring video. I'm looking for ways to heal myself, and this helped. You're serving a great need for moms. Thank you.

***

I love that so many people reached out today and prayed and sent positive thoughts to me. I never realized a group so wonderful was out here! I sat still, I waited it out, my ALO did whatever he does, and I survived. I didn't enable today!

Look how this group helps each of us face yucky days. Look at the love and support. I am so humbled and grateful for you as I cry tears of relief.

As you can see, my efforts to help moms of addicted loved ones, help others. What if these moms hadn't found help or support? Where would they be today?

What about you? If you could see your future impact on others, what would that look like? Imagine your Boon coming true.

CLOSE YOUR GAP DAY 5: COUNT YOUR COST

Today you'll write a fictitious letter to yourself from someone you want to serve as you work toward your Boon. Seeing the reality of the reward will help you push past the fear and create your legacy.

Next, write a fictitious letter from your addicted loved one to you. Be honest about what you'd like to hear from your child.

In each letter, pretend to see the future. These letters will help you overcome the fear of changing. This powerful process is called an imaginary impact.

Now faith is the assurance of things hoped for, the conviction of things not seen.
—Hebrews 11:1 (NRSV)

These letters are only the beginning. Imagine influencing hundreds, thousands, and millions of people. What if they're waiting for you to show them the way? It's time to stop focusing on your fears and find faith.

From the All-Mighty Mom Tribe

Lucretia

My Boon is to see moms of incarcerated children get unstuck. My son ended up in jail and then prison for two years. Since his recent release, he's doing great things with his life. I praise God and want to serve other moms because I know first-hand how important it is to heal. Here are my two letters:

Dear Lucretia,

Thank you for guiding me on this difficult journey. When my son went to prison, I couldn't sleep and thought I'd have a stroke because my blood pressure was so high. I thought I was going to die that day.

You helped me understand the jail and prison process, so I had realistic expectations. You shared the terms and the politics, so I understood what my son was going through. You calmed my fears, taught me how to take care of my health, and coached me to overcome my worry.

Because of your help, I eat healthier and have been able to lose twenty pounds, bringing my blood pressure down. Now I'm off my hypertension meds. My son is in jail and not using, so I've been able to build a better relationship with him too.

I appreciate you serving in this ministry.

A Thankful Mom

Dear Mom,

Thank you for working on your recovery instead of trying to fix me.

During my active addiction, I was angry because you wouldn't give me what I wanted. I thought you didn't love me, but I was wrong. You loved me enough to believe in me and empower me to take control of my life. You loved me enough to let go of your shame and guilt and the chaos I was causing.

You showed me my life mattered to you, but you couldn't fix me. You gave me hope there was a better life available if I chose it.

Your child

PART TWO

Flawless Hope Anatomy

Claim Your Promise

*The most important person to
keep your promises to is yourself.*

—Anonymous

I n Unveiling, Part One of this book, you shared your present story, created your Boon, admitted you're the enemy, seized your saboteur, and discovered the cost of getting hacked.

In this section, we're going to unlock the secrets to finding hope, dissect what hope looks like, and discover your hope.

HOPE stands for Having Only Positive Expectations. Unfortunately, the lies and years of unhealthy attitudes and choices make it difficult to see anything positive. Every time our child demonstrates a glimmer of healing, relapse steals our hope. Statistics regarding relapses ending in overdose deaths confirm our negative expectations.

I never imagined my son and daughter-in-law would be in recovery for thirty-one months and stay married through it. When they were living in the misery of addiction three years ago, we couldn't envision them finding a way out of the storm.

One day, I said to my husband, "What is the best-case scenario for everyone—our children, grandchildren, and us?"

He shrugged.

"Would you say Ryan and Angelika finding sobriety, rebuilding their lives, staying married, parenting their children, and leading productive lives?"

"Yeah, right." Sarcasm laced his reply.

"I know it's hard to fathom, based on the past, but if it's the best situation, we have to keep our eyes on that prize. We must pray for that outcome. See it, believe it, and pray for it."

I had never believed full recovery to be a possibility. On that day, I began to embrace this positive expectation. I envisioned it and believed it could happen. My son and daughter-in-law's healing topped every prayer.

Slowly, I noticed God working miracles. At first, the changes were small, like he and his wife showing up for counseling appointments with their children. Though they were often compromised, they were on time, and we could tell they cared. Each day brought another little change, until the little things started adding up to something big.

I had proven I couldn't control their actions. But I could command my response. I could choose to stay calm, pray, and love them through the storm.

Was it easy?

No.

Did I fail repeatedly?

Yes. I couldn't look at them most days.

So how did I do it?

I turned my focus to trusting God with my future and my son and daughter-in-law's healing.

Moving from Negative to Positive Expectations

Ralph Waldo Emerson said, "You become what you think about all day long." We have the ability to remold ourselves by transforming our minds.

Did you know memory works in two directions—backward and forward? The latest brain science confirms imagining the future uses many of the same brain areas as remembering the past. Your brain activates the hippocampus and medial temporal lobe for all mental time travel—when visiting the past or going into the unknown.[11] Each time you think about something in the future, whether you worry or see positivity, you remember your future.

Focusing on fear produces anxiety. Focusing on the possibility our children will die of an overdose robs us of our hope. Refocusing on our recovery and praying for a best-case scenario restores it.

Another method of transformation can be found in Dr. Caroline Leaf's book, *Cleaning Up Your Mental Mess: 5 Simple, Scientifically Proven Steps to Reduce Anxiety, Stress, and Toxic Thinking*. Using the principles of neuroplasticity, Dr. Leaf provides a plan to catch and alter our thoughts and reactions before they become toxic neural networks and habits.

You can overcome your negative thoughts, learning to manage your mind in any number of ways. With intentionality, we can find resources to help us learn the skills necessary to change our response to the chaos and take control of our life. With practice, we can learn how to HOPE—Have Only Positive Expectations.

First, we need to make a promise—a promise to ourselves that we will lean into learning. The most important step in fulfilling your promise is to know why you're in recovery and the purpose of the promise. Why are you taking time to read this book and implement changes in your life?

CLOSE YOUR GAP DAY 6: CLAIM YOUR PROMISE

If you want to claim your promise and win, you need to clarify your why.

Below are several reasons we choose to recover:

- to learn how to let go of the fear, negative thoughts, and shame so we can live instead of simply existing
- to embrace our feelings
- to understand and acknowledge our trauma
- to establish better relationships with friends and family
- to recapture our identity and purpose
- to sleep, eat, and cope in healthier ways
- to use our gifts to build the Kingdom
- to grow in faith and spirituality

Michelle's Why

I must recover so I can write *Unhackable Moms of Addicted Loved Ones* to continue empowering one million moms into recovery by 2025.

The questions below will help you commit to making yourself a priority.

1. Why are you choosing recovery? List your reasons.

   _____

   _____

2. How will you promise to change? What promises will you make to yourself? List them.

   _____

   _____

3. Find an accountability partner, someone who will be
   your truth teller if you get stuck. Who will that be?
   How do you want that person to hold you accountable?

Here are a few examples:

- Learn how to love your child despite the addiction.
- Embrace empathy statements instead of "fix-it"
  statements.
- Learn the BLESS Method of communicating and the
  PEACE Method of listening. (See Appendix B.)
- No longer pay your child's bills, car payments, or
  living expenses.
- Allow your child to take the consequences of his/her
  actions no matter how serious they are.
- Spend time every week reading about addiction and
  how to keep boundaries. (See reading recommendations
  in Appendix C.)
- See a therapist twice a month.
- Create a Daily Affirmation Chart.
- Talk to a recovering addict who's been sober for two
  years or more. Ask that person the questions you want
  to ask your addicted child.

Sign and Date your Promise to Change.

_____   _____

Addicted loved ones recover every day. They make a promise to stay true to themselves. You can too. Moms who make
promises to themselves heal.

Notes from the All-Mighty Mom Tribe

Darra

My dream is a unified family which includes all members relating to each other with respect. Together, we will celebrate victories and comfort disappointments. We are grateful for family; no one is left out. I believe this will happen in the next few years. I desire to share this success story with my community/universe to mend other broken families.

***

Lucretia

My why and my passion—To encourage and equip other women on their journey of self-care in whatever season they are going through.

My promise—I claim growth in my life-coaching business by speaking and coaching 5,000 ladies by 2025. I want to inspire moms of addicted loved ones to become unstuck and take the next step in their own recovery. God has promised me an abundant life, living above the mediocre. I am a promise person, and I will focus on God's promises.

***

Brooke

My dream is to travel, spend beautiful and meaningful girls' weekends, love my husband well, be a good mom and a better step-monster (or stepmom), and have a meaningful career that pays my bills.

***

Joshua's Story

Written by his mother, Lucretia.

With tissues tucked neatly in my purse just in case, I sat in my car trying to collect myself before entering the Sebastian County Jail. It was time to see Joshua, my youngest son, and let him know things were going to change. I had tried everything, and nothing was working, so now, it was up to him. Between November 2017 and June 2019, Joshua had been arrested seven times. The last time had been on June 7 for theft, and the judge set no bond.

I inhaled deeply, opened my door, and got out, pushing past my fears. The humidity of the hot Arkansas July day slapped me into reality. This wasn't a dream. I was going to visit my son in jail, a place I'd never been before. I didn't know what to expect. Joshua was the first of my seven children to be in jail.

I swallowed hard. "Why are you here, Lucretia?" Silently, I answered myself, "To tell Joshua I love and care about him and that I can't help him anymore. He must help himself."

I entered through the glass doors into a cold waiting room with several metal chairs. A man and a woman looked up when I entered but then looked away. I approached the window.

"Yes?" a man said.

"I'm here to see my son, Joshua Talley."

"Driver's license."

I pulled out my wallet and handed him my license.

After giving it a quick look, he copied it and handed it back. "Through that door over there," he said, motioning to my left. "When the door in the waiting room buzzes, you can go in."

The first door opened into the waiting room. The sound of it closing echoed off the stark floors.

Alone, I sat in the first of two rows of metal chairs. Joshua's name with the appointment time flashed on the old TV monitor in the corner of the room. I still had five minutes.

Beige concrete walls stared back at me as I waited. The room smelled of fading hope and lost dreams. I swallowed the deep guttural moan that wanted to escape. It formed a lump in the fringe of my throat.

To focus on staying calm, I read the signs lining the walls.

"Women cannot wear shirts that show any amount of their stomach, chest, or shoulders.

"This includes spaghetti strap T-shirts, belly shirts, halter tops, and similar tops. While men also are not allowed to wear low-cut V-neck shirts, women should be extra-conservative in this regard, as even mildly low-cut shirts may inadvertently be too revealing.

"Both men and women should take caution to ensure shirts and tops are in good repair when visiting their incarcerated loved one.

"Ripped, torn, or frayed clothing may be deemed unacceptable, as they may reveal too much of the individual's body (even if done so unintentionally).

"One last thing to note regarding shirts and tops is that they need to be completely opaque. In other words, visitors should ensure their undershirts and/or bras are not visible through their overshirt or top at all."

I shivered, wishing I had brought a jacket.

The buzz of the metal door startled me. Standing, I moved across the "room" feeling like I was having an out-of-body experience.

The visitation room was larger, like an abandoned storage room with a tiled floor and more beige walls. To my right sat cubicles with metal chairs facing PLEXIGLAS® windows and TV monitors. A black receiver, like one from a 1970s-style phone, hung on the right side of each cubicle. The room looked like something out of a thriller movie.

I sat in one cubicle chair and faced the dark monitor. My heart flapped like bird wings. What was I going to say?

Suddenly, the screen lit up, and Joshua stared back at me. "Hi, Mom. It's so good to see you." His face was fuller than the last time I had seen him. The dark circles were gone, and his pupils were normal.

I couldn't find the words. What was I supposed to talk about? How's it going in there? How's the food? Are you sleeping well? All those questions moms ask about safety and self-care didn't feel right. But that was all I had.

"Are you sleeping well?"

"The first three weeks were tough. I had to sleep on the floor with no pillow or a blanket. But I'm getting used to it now."

I choked back a sob. "I'm glad you're not homeless anymore, but are you," I paused for a moment as I looked for the right word, "okay?"

He nodded. "Don't worry about me." He looked down. "I'm sorry for what I've put you through." Tears filled his eyes.

I believed him.

"Everything is going to be okay, but . . ." he said.

"What?"

"Could you bring me a Bible?"

Tears ran down my cheeks. "Of course."

"You have to give it to the chaplain. That's the only way they'll allow it."

I wiped my tears with the back of my hand. "Sure."

"Don't cry, Mom."

"Joshua, I'll bring the Bible, but I can't help you anymore. We've tried everything. God has plans for you, but you must do your part. We can't help you get well if you don't want to get well."

He nodded.

Our allotted twenty minutes ran out. I had to leave. "I'll schedule an appointment to come next week so I can bring a Bible."

"Thank you."

As I left that room, with him at my back and on the other side of a PLEXIGLAS, it was never more obvious that there was nothing I could do for him. This journey was his, and only he could fight his battle.

I reached into my purse and balled the tissues in my fist. By the time I reached my car, the tissues were soaked with years of tears.

DAY 7

Inventory Your Value

If you hear a voice within you say, "You cannot paint,"
then by all means, paint, and that voice will be silenced.

—Vincent Van Gogh

Years ago, as I was writing a memoir for a young woman, I had the opportunity to pitch her story to a literary agent. "Don't spend your time writing that book. It will never sell," he said. "What else are you working on?"

His abrupt response caught me off guard. I felt as if he'd slapped me across the face. I had spent hours interviewing the author, and we had chunks of the book written and recorded. It was a powerful story.

At the time, I hadn't yet published, so I didn't understand the industry. The agent did, and I trusted and respected his opinion. I shared a few of my other projects with him, and he encouraged me to write those books instead.

Later, as I reflected on our meeting, I wondered how he really knew what would sell and what wouldn't. I didn't like someone else instantly deciding the future of my project.

He barely heard my pitch. He didn't know the whole story. He hadn't heard about the miracles that would bring other people hope.

Unfortunately, I didn't know how to publish a book without him, so I abandoned that project and continued writing my other books. For months, I read about writing and followed marketing experts to learn inside publishing tips and tricks. I joined blogs and made friends with other authors who knew the industry. I figured out how to self-publish and launched two books. They became Amazon best sellers.

Shortly afterward, I returned to the young woman and said, "Your story will change lives. I feel called to write it. I've learned how to publish and market books on my own. We can do it without an agent. Do you want to give it another shot?"

She did.

Her book, *Fractured Not Broken*, has sold more copies and changed more lives than any of my previous books. It's optioned for a movie. We get fan mail often.

Her book was my baby. I believed in the power of her story to bring hope to other people. I knew its value.

Even after your child is an adult, he or she is still your baby. You birthed him. You know his value and see his potential. Unlike others who only see the addict, you see beneath the surface, beyond the disease. You see your child without the enemy attached to his brain. Though fading, you still have hopes and dreams for him. You know his heart.

That's one thing that makes this journey difficult. We want others to see our children like we do, but the symptoms of addiction clothe them in a dark fog. Even those who love them struggle to see beneath their blood-shot eyes and emaciated bodies.

God has a purpose for your child's life. We don't know what that is, but we find peace when we realize God loves our children more than we do.

Discovering Our True Value

Our children need us to stay connected. But if staying connected means you must fix your child's problems, take the consequences of his actions, and allow him to overstep boundaries, then you may need to work with a therapist. Fixers must unlearn deeply ingrained family dynamics. Working with a therapist can shed light on where you're stuck.

Joel Osteen said, "God knows your value; He sees your potential. You may not understand everything you are going through right now. But hold

> Until you value yourself, you won't value your time.
> —**Unknown**

your head up high, knowing that God is in control, and He has a great plan and purpose for your life."[12]

On Day Twenty-Three, we'll explore deeper the need for boundaries, but before we can create effective limits, we must embrace our value. We've already spent time recognizing this for our children. It's time to accept it for ourselves.

Many moms of ALOs blame themselves for their child's disease. We make a list of all the things we could have done differently and replay their lives looking for our mistakes. If we contemplate our role in our child's bad choices too long, we begin to mimic their behavior. The only difference is our child has become our addiction.

One of the best ways to overcome this is to create a new list. Rather than remembering mistakes, things every human does, catalog every moment of value you bring. When we recognize our gifts and talents and begin to use them to make the world a better place, we become Unhackable. Each day, make a list of every person you helped, each stranger who smiled because of you—these people see your value. God created you with beauty and purpose; He values you.

CLOSE YOUR GAP DAY 7: INVENTORY YOUR VALUE

Before others can value us, we must value ourselves. On this day, I encourage you to inventory your value.

Take inventory of those things that make you feel responsible for your child's addiction. Journal these questions:

- Why do I believe I am responsible for this problem in my child?
- What should I have done differently?
- Is my child's addiction a parenting error?
- How can I release myself from this guilt?

Take inventory of your gifts, talents, and treasures, those things you can use to help others. List them.

Make a list of your gifts, talents, and treasures before addiction hacked you. Value and pay attention to the little things you love to do. It might be tough to find those things, but what we focus on, we see. It will take practice to find them.

Take inventory of those things you're doing well. Look closely. Keep noticing.

Notes from the All-Mighty Mom Tribe

Brooke

I love to laugh and dance. I can be very uninhibited. I have wisdom to speak into hard situations. I am very childlike and enjoy being around children. I have curiosity about the world and few restrictions on how I explore that. I am always learning and growing.

***

Sandy

God has blessed me with many gifts. I am an encourager who notices the potential in others. I am a teacher, counselor, effective communicator, and a leader. I serve others through generosity and hospitality by using my sewing, baking, and knitting skills. I love to learn and strive to grow closer to God each day.

***

Teresa

I am grateful God has given me the gift of being a kind, caring, and empathetic person, a trustworthy friend, and faithful believer.

***

Lucretia

I thank God for His grace and love. He has gifted me with a deep love for people and discernment in helping them see the positive in life. I am a teacher, coach, speaker, organizer, leader, and empathetic friend with a soft, teachable spirit for the Lord. God is awesome. He shows His attributes and character through each of us!

Track Your Progress

Imperfect action is better than perfect inaction.
—Harry S. Truman

Have you ever had an idea to create, invent, or do something only to discover that somebody else stole your idea before you accomplished your dream? So often what we envision for our lives never materializes. We hesitate and procrastinate. We believe the lies: *I don't have the experience, or the knowledge, or the time and confidence to accomplish that dream.* We think, *I need to flesh out my idea first. I need to gather information first. I need to pay off my car first.* We make excuses. Then one day, we wake up, and we discover we waited too long.

Change isn't easy for anyone, but there is a secret to accomplishing something new, to embracing change. By breaking the dream down into little steps, we take the fear out of change.

Our ALOSs present another compelling reason to embrace change. Why should our addicted loved ones change if they see their mom unwilling to do the work? We need to take the first step, imperfect and uncertain as it may be, even if we know we'll make mistakes.

My eighty-nine-year-old father recently moved into an independent living home that he loves. After four weeks, he knew almost every resident's name. He also started a comedy hour/sing-along with his new neighbors.

People are amazed Dad is so sharp. He said he doesn't feel old inside.

Maybe you can relate. Though we age a bit every day, often we don't feel older in our minds.

I encouraged Dad to try something new because he didn't seem intimidated about most things, but also, selfishly, I wanted a keepsake from him. I created it in my mind first, then shared it with him.

"I think you should start a podcast." He loved Toastmasters and embraced speaking. People often told him he had a radio voice. "It would be an awesome legacy for your children and grandchildren. Even your great-great-granchildren, whom you'll never meet, will be able to listen to your stories."

He didn't answer. I could tell he was letting the idea sink in, so I didn't say much more.

The next day, he leaned in and whispered, "I'm going to do it."

"What?"

"Start a podcast. I'll call it *Minutes with Maurice*."

For almost a week afterward, I coached him on how to use his phone and the Anchor App to create and publish stories. He writes his prose long hand on paper and reads them. In one day, he lost recordings, stuttered, paused for too long, and messed up dates. We deleted sections and started over. Sometimes he can't find the STOP button on the app. Other times, he records a new story only to discover that the audio had disappeared.

Nevertheless, he continues to push forward. Today, he has accumulated three published short personal stories.

He has many questions that can't be answered: How long will I do this? Where will I find stories? How many should I record in a week? Who will listen?

I encourage him by saying, "For now, keep making forward progress, and your ideas will ebb and flow. What you're doing now might be different two months from now because you're going to learn 'on the grow.' You can't anticipate what you're going to learn. The best experience is reflective—understanding what went well, what went wrong, and readjusting. Keep an open mind. We can't predict how this will transition or if it will. All you can do is continue to take imperfect action."

Let's break down this process and look at the steps Dad has taken up until now:

1. He was inspired with an idea.
2. He assessed his interest and researched the idea.
3. He found a teacher, coach, or mentor.
4. He created a mental plan.
5. He tried the idea and failed.
6. He tried the idea again and made mistakes.
7. He learned from the mistakes.
8. He repeated a similar adjusted step.
9. He published his first podcast.
10. He created a list of writing prompts.
11. He got into a rhythm of writing and posting and committed to publishing two episodes a week.
12. He repeated the process.

Imagine how many followers he will accumulate over time. More importantly, consider his legacy, the lives he will change, and the influence he will make.

We can't predict the results of implementing something new, but in Dad's case, his action inspires me. I, as well as the rest of the family, will cherish each one of his recordings.

If we don't take time to notice and celebrate each little step, we can easily give up. Find someone who understands your Boon so you can celebrate all the little wins together.

Fear is wetting your pants. **Courage** is doing what you're supposed to do with wet pants. You don't feel **capable** until you are **committed** to doing it afraid, and you don't gain **confidence** until you feel capable. You must be able to embrace these 4 Cs to win.

—Dan Sullivan

An Example from the Garden

Little seeds in our garden start out as the tiniest speck of hope. Seeds grow into seedlings that grow into stalks that grow into buds and bloom into flowers. This process doesn't happen overnight, but if we plant that seed in the right environment, nurture it, and watch it grow, we appreciate every little change we see. We can help it move a bit quicker by planting it in the most productive place and pulling the weeds that sprout up nearby. The plant will absorb more nutrients and sunshine, which help it grow.

But each plant has its timetable. If we plant a redwood tree seedling, the growth process will take much longer, but the tree will grow much larger and exist longer too.

Your idea might be smaller in comparison to someone else's Boon, but it doesn't mean your Boon is any less significant. Moving forward in your progress and appreciating every small step is all that matters.

I encourage you to look at your Boon in the same way. Plant your idea or dream seed in an environment like the All-Mighty Mom Tribe where we'll celebrate the little steps and fight the weedy setbacks with you.

The progress of little steps is easy to miss. You won't see it as clearly as your setbacks. Unless you watch for them, you'll only see the mini-steps when you look back.

In his book *The Gap and the Gain: The High Achievers' Guide to Happiness, Confidence, and Success,* Dan Sullivan said, "The way to measure your progress is backward against where you started, not against your ideal."

In *Unhackable,* Kary Oberbrunner tells us that tracking our progress is simple and necessary. We need to celebrate progress, regardless of size. This helps us establish a deep root. The root needs to be strong enough to support your Boon.

Tracking my progress has become a gratitude poem to myself.

As you work toward your recovery and your Boon, track your progress. But before you begin tracking, it helps to identify some of the steps you will take.

Many items from the list of promises on Day 6 could be little steps, as would any of these:

- Join a support meeting.
- Practice meditation or mindfulness.
- Exercise.
- Participate in a Bible study.
- Send positive memes to addicted child.
- Learn motivational interviewing techniques. (Appendix A.)
- Research recovery and rehab options.

- Spend time with other family members without talking about your ALO.
- Hire a coach or mentor.
- Join the All-Mighty Mom Tribe for continued support, accountability, and inspiration.

CLOSE YOUR GAP DAY 8: TRACK YOUR PROGRESS

List every small step you've made toward achieving your Boon, including reading this book. Keep a log of every little step you take toward your goal so you can see your progress and feel inspired to continue.

Sample Chart

Date   Activity

_____   _____
_____   _____
_____   _____

Have you ever had a goal or Boon before and given up because you didn't see results soon enough? After today's mission, what new commitments will you make going forward so you don't abandon this Boon?

If you knew your Boon was guaranteed if you didn't quit, would you keep putting in the effort? Why or why not?

Having a self-care plan might be another baby step toward accomplishing your Boon. List five actions you can add to your self-care routine. Which action will you take in the next twenty-four hours?

Notes from the All-Mighty Mom Tribe

Michelle

My self-care routine includes reciting positive affirmations, visualizing my dream, eating one more serving of veggies every day, reading fifteen pages in addiction/self-help books every week, spending fifteen minutes in the Word every day, and doing one thing every day that scares me.

***

Lucretia

Day trips are part of my self-care routine. I call them adventure days. I go on a walk or hike, eat at a new restaurant, pack a picnic, and have lunch by the water. I will be honest with my feelings and triggers and ask my husband to hold me accountable, pray with me, and remind me to breathe. I want to display positive energy and schedule a massage.

***

Brooke

My husband is my safe spot. He grounds me and helps me think rationally. I exercise every day, walking 15,000 steps most days. I hike, kayak, water ski, and spend lots of time with girlfriends. I meditate, go to Bible study, and pray.

***

Tracking Your Progress from a Different Perspective

Once our addicted loved ones get into recovery, they, too, find power in tracking their recovery progress. It helps bring healing. Below is Crystal Waltman's illustration of Day 8. Crystal is an Unhackable Coach and the author of *Quitting to Win.*

Ninety days sober. Is this what a baby feels like? My skin is different. I rub my arm and snap the rubber band on my wrist. Yep. I'm still alive. I wiggle my toes and fingers. No headache, no blank space. I flutter my eyes, grateful for yesterday. Today's a new day. I sit on the side of my bed, take a deep breath, point, and flex my feet, raise my arms over head and sway back and forth. I have so many new unanswered thoughts. "How will I find my words today? How will I find my new voice? What will I sound like? Will people like me? Will I be funny?"

Quickly, I snap back to the present. "What others think of me is not my business. I don't have to worry anymore about what others think."

I recite what I remember from the laminated morning prayer card, "God release me from the bondage of self."

"Progress not perfection," I remind myself as I finish my morning routine.

Ninety-plus degrees and a bright sun beating through my windshield has warmed my car. I glance in the rearview mirror, give myself a smile, notice my eyes are less puffy and my skin is not dry today. "Use the mirror for self-reflection and love, not looking back." The words run through my head. "I can't move forward if I am looking in the rearview mirror," I say out loud.

I park in front of the church, put up the reflective sunshade, and step into the heat. Taking a deep breath, I check my book to make sure the one-dollar bills are there.

"What will happen tomorrow?" No. Don't go there. Be in the moment. The car chirps as I click the car remote. The sound brings the satisfaction of completion. I got here, which is the hard part. The rest of the day will be ok.

With just enough courage, I walk into the church and head toward the gathering room. My heart beats a little faster.

Ninety days ago, I did not know a soul. Not even my own. Today, I walk in looking forward to seeing my sponsor and a few women whom I have taken a liking to. I am greeted with a hug and a ticket.

A bag of mixed emotions, I inch my way into the room filled with women. After a few more steps, I glance around the room. Smiles, as well as sad faces, greet me, but we all know every expression is valid; we have been taught to own our feelings. One thing I like about the meeting is the room of emotions is unapologetic; we all stand strong in our feelings.

In the next room, kids play and mothers coo their little ones to sleep. I left my little at home today so I could have extra time to connect. A low chatter fills the room like a bunch of hens.

Today is special. I did it by taking one day at time. One minute at a time. I am ninety days sober. Today I track my progress. I'm celebrating ninety meetings in ninety days with hugs, a medallion, and cake. I can't get arrested for eating cake.

Today, I will have the courage to speak. I swallow a lump in my throat, nervously.

I sit in the same chair every Friday, or as close as I can to the middle of the room. Not in the front row. That is reserved for the veterans. I am not there yet. We leave the back row for the hiding newbies. In the middle row of folding chairs,

I set my book down, smell the coffee, and realize how far I have come.

After the arrivals greet one another, the meeting's sober birthday countdown begins. "One day or twenty-four hours," my friend and facilitator, Sandy, calls out.

I remember when that was me, crying shamefully and plagued with guilt. One woman sneaks up from the back row. Boy, I feel her pain. I nod to myself and make a mental note to give her a hug after the meeting.

"One month," Sandy announces.

A familiar face stands up. Wait! What? She has more time than I do. She is at one month again? Why? What happened? I sit in shock. Her courage radiates throughout the room as she takes the chip and leans in for a hug.

Meeting hugs are like nothing I have ever experienced before. They are heartfelt and sincere. Not socially polite, not a have-to-because-you're-my-family-member-and-hugs-are-a -part-of-the-protocol. These deep hugs transfer energy, as a drop of water revives a cactus. They bring tides that roll over me like the next monsoon season.

"Ninety days," Sandy announces.

I stand up. Time stops. I sweat, my face flushes. Focus on Sandy. Find Sandy's face. Sandy smiles warmly at me. It is ok; I can walk forward. I approach her with open arms, and she gives me the tightest hug. I take the medallion and a tear rolls down my cheek. As I return to my seat, I think, "You're okay. Just be."

I am alive. I have made five new friends who have shared their deepest secrets. I have a loving relationship with my sponsor. I can leave the house with my daughter and return when I say I am going to return. I don't have headaches. My body aches are disappearing. The thoughts of wanting to go "out of my mind" have left. I can be sober and function.

I spend the morning on self-care and the latter part of the day focusing on being a present mother and wife. Today, I want to live. For today, I am at peace.

DAY 9

Strengthen Your Posture

Failure and setbacks are ingredients for a great success story.
My setback was a blessing!
I survived what was meant to destroy me.
I came back like a boss—fabulous, wiser,
and stronger than ever.

—A Recovering Addict

The mobile phone rings. A strange number appears on the caller ID. Our heart skips a beat. Is this *the call,* the one that informs us our child overdosed? We answer, adrenaline racing. It's the county jail with a collect call from our child.

"Will you accept the charges?"

How could we not? We enter our credit card information and hold our breath.

"Mom?"

"Yes?"

"You have to get me out of here. Please, I'm begging you. I have the money. I'll pay you back. I'll sell things."

We never imagined our children would end up behind bars. Our children aren't criminals. They're sick. We think, *They haven't hurt anyone but themselves.*

The first time they're in jail, we might bail them out because we have preconceived notions of what jail is like. We've watched plenty of movies that show hardened criminals with bulging biceps beating on the weak inmates, raping them, and smuggling in drugs. Our first instincts are to rescue our children from the trauma we're sure they will experience.

We bail them out only to see them end up in jail again. This time, a little more seasoned about the reality of jail, we feel relief because we know living on the street could be the other alternative.

"Mom, you have to listen to me. This time is different. I promise. Bail me out, and I'll pay you back. Please don't leave me here."

With each arrest, we learn more about the chronic and progressive nature of an SUD. We also discover society doesn't love our children like we do. Desperate people will do desperate things, illegal things. We feel shame and embarrassment because we believe our children reflect our success—or lack of success. We think they embody our parenting flaws.

Perfect moms, perfect parents—they don't exist. That concept is a myth.

People trapped in the throes of addiction have upside down logic and unhealthy reasoning skills. We can't rationalize with them, so eventually we learn it's healthier not to engage in the angry battles. It's better to listen and respond with calm patience. It won't be easy. But as we reset our goals to better lead ourselves in this situation, and guard our self-care, we quickly learn using the BLESS and PEACE methods of listening work much better. (Find these methods in Appendix B.)

How Will You Strengthen Your Posture?

Expect setbacks and possible relapses with your ALO. We can't stop them, but we can prepare ourselves for them. How will you stay strong in your recovery and not get sucked back into hopelessness? How will you stay positive when family members don't support your recovery endeavors? Many family members won't understand why you refuse to bail your child out of jail. They will judge when you won't let him live with you instead of wandering the streets. When guilt presses or your spouse wants you to handle a situation differently, who will you lean on to help you stay focused on your self-care?

Resiliency can be learned. Identify your feelings and how you'd rather be feeling, then draw on past experiences when you showed resiliency, that decision that allowed you to feel something positive. Search your memory for those actions and situations that brought hope and optimism. Donating time to a worthy cause or becoming active in something you're passionate about can redirect your energy and create positivity in a way you can control.

You can also reframe negative thought patterns. One way is using the ABCDE cognitive behavior model used in therapy.

A. Name the **ADVERSITY**.

B. Examine negative **BELIEFS** you have about your situation.

C. Consider the **CONSEQUENCES** (on your behavior and emotions and how you feel about yourself) of having that belief.

D. **DISPUTE** those beliefs and offer alternative explanations to yourself.

E. **ENERGIZE** or realize a new **EFFECT,** a new line of thinking about the adversity.

Let's look at this model using a fictitious, but probable, situation.

A. **Adversity**. Our children have SUDs, possibly combined with a mental health disorder, and we can't make them stop using.

B. **Belief.** We've faced this adversity for a long time, and the problem isn't getting better. Each declaration of recovery has been followed by relapse. We've begun to let fear drive our beliefs. Many drugs are laced with fentanyl now, increasing the overdose incidences. We believe our children will be taken by death, jail, or prison.

C. **Consequences.** Worry consumes us. We can't sleep, we're anxious, and our blood pressure is elevated. We've lost money, family and friend relationships have suffered, and our displaced guilt keeps us in the vicious cycle of enablers.

D. **Dispute.** We choose to disagree with our negative beliefs about our children dying or ending up in jail. As we focus on developing a new thought pattern, we talk to recovering addicts. People recover every day, so we focus on that. Searching for the hope will aid in building our resilience. We will interview a recovered addict, preferably someone with over two years of recovery. We will ask them to honestly tell their story, even the worst details. The fact they found a successful and happy life, even though they were terribly sick like our children, will help dispute those negative beliefs. We will find out what their mother did to help them and learn from their success.

E. **Energize.** Find a new line of thinking. Instead of focusing on things we can't control, we will focus our energy on what we can. We can spend our energy on a one-sheet resource page, collecting names, phone numbers, and locations of possible rehab options for our children. We can visit these places, check their reviews, and examine funding options, such as insurance, Medicaid, and free facilities. Professionals in our area can give us recommendations. We can research the idea of an intervention. Knowledge gives us a feeling of control.

Having this sense of control strengthens our postures and fosters hope. Unfortunately, we fail when we continually try to regulate what's happening to our children. The ABCDE method helps us find positive things to focus on in our lives. It allows us to draw on our resilience and let go of things beyond our control or our ability to influence. Finding another course of action, like creating a resource page, relieves some of the unpleasant emotions of our difficult situation.

You don't need to solve your child's problem to feel some success.

In our All-Mighty Mom Tribe, we lean on each other for honest, authentic connections. We're all moms of addicted loved ones who understand each other's plight. Our stories may be different, but our emotions and fears are similar. We

> Seek hope in at least one positive act, and you may begin to see a glimmer of light you had missed before.
> **—Betty J. Edie,**
> *Embracing the Light*

feel seen and heard. This virtual safe place allows us to share our problems head-on with no filter. We talk about the true terribleness of each story. Sometimes we cry. We actively listen. We are engaged and empathetic. We have open, vulnerable conversations, which help us feel less hopeless. Our group meets several times a week via video conferencing. Moms find our group valuable for healing because we build authentic connections and focus on healthier emotional well-beings.

Enthusiasm Builds Hope

Enthusiasm means possessed by God. When we're enthusiastic, we're aware of our relationship with God. When our loved ones relapse or continue in their battle with addiction, it can be difficult to find enthusiasm. If we have something positive to focus on, like our Boon, it helps, especially when we see that our Boon comes from above. We begin to realize our Boon is greater than us.

Our new focus doesn't take away the sting, the fear, and the grief of having a sick child, but we don't allow ourselves to stay stuck in our grief. We feel the loss, embrace it, and then bounce back because we know God counts on us to carry through with our dream—our Boon—to benefit others.

Staying enthusiastic helps strengthen our postures and sustain our hope.

CLOSE YOUR GAP DAY 9: STRENGTHEN YOUR POSTURE

For today's assignment, answer these questions:

- What are three practical ways you can strengthen your hope right now?
- What if no one supports you or your Boon? How will you feel? And how will you respond?
- How will you treat your Boon differently now that you know it has been entrusted to you from above?
- How will you and your spouse build a united and supportive front?

- From this day forward, with your Boon in mind, will you make a conscious commitment to turn your set-backs into comebacks?

_____Yes   _____No

let this fight become the fuel to strengthen your posture?

_____Yes   _____No

operate with enthusiasm?

_____Yes   _____No

From the All-Mighty Mom Tribe

Sandy

My husband, Scott, has been my rock and constant voice of reason. He has listened to me sob and spew my hurt-filled rants. He has held me and been calm. We have worked through boundaries and searched for answers and help. He doesn't say a lot, but his faith is rock solid, and his reliance on God is unwavering.

***

Lucretia

We always knew with a large family there would be ups and downs, so we say, "Are you still holding my hand?" We picture the two of us holding hands, walking down a train track. He walks on one side, and I walk on the other. If we are united on the same track, God will get us through whatever.

***

Tammy

I plan to redirect my energy by

- using the Peloton
- spending twenty minutes a day in a quiet room, listening and talking to the Lord
- staying out of cop/detective mode. I will stop looking for things my son is doing wrong and start celebrating and praising him for all he's doing right
- managing time better so I can spend time doing things that bring me joy

***

Brooke

I plan to redirect my energy with exercise, fellowship with friends, spiritual practice, listening to my husband, and enjoying others in the family.

DAY 10

Create Your Boon Road Map

The obstacles of your past can become the gateways that lead to new beginnings.

—Ralph Blum

O nce an addicted loved one decides to get sober and commits to living a life without abusing mind-altering substances, they unintentionally create a Boon. They might not call it a Boon, but we see it in the word's definition: a gift the hero receives as a reward for achieving her goals. It's your truest longing, your greatest ache. It can be different things for different heroes, but what all Boons have in common is that this gift is of great value.

Let's look at what our child's Boon might be for himself and compare it to the Boon we have for them.

Ask your child this question: "If you could wave a magic wand that took away all your troubles, what would your life look like?" You might be surprised at their answer.

Several Tribe moms asked their recovering sons this question. Here are a couple answers:

- "Why are you asking me that question? You don't want to know the answer." This left his mother wondering, but she didn't press him.

- Lucretia's son, Joshua, said, "I wouldn't wave a wand because nothing worth having comes easy. When the good things come, if you don't have perspective on how bad things can be, you won't appreciate how good things are."

These obviously aren't the Boons these two moms had created for their sons. The exercise demonstrates, once again, we can't create a life for our children. Part of the problem lies in the fact their Boons were created unintentionally. As they walk forward, they struggle. Though they've set out to be sober, they don't see past today. If we don't create our Boon road map, we could fall in right behind them.

What if you had a magic wand? What would your life look like?

Unfortunately, magic wands don't exist. Achieving a Boon takes dedication, time, planning, and patience. Joy comes after we do the work. But if we never take time to imagine what our Boon life looks like, it will probably never happen. We must act—take a step—even if we have doubts about the Boon-life image we've created. Each step we take, the road becomes clearer. Our Boon story may take turns we never imagined, but creating the story helps us know where to start.

In our journey toward our Boon, each next step requires imperfect action. Most people don't like that advice. We want to be sure of the outcome before we move. But clarity comes only after we take action. In the beginning, the way forward is never smooth, clear, or obvious. The more steps you take, the more committed you feel, the more capable you become, and the more clearly you will see the next step.

Once we begin to determine our Boon, we'll know what step to take. We can distinguish between the distractions (hacking moments) and divine interruptions.

Let me illustrate this concept for you. Several weeks ago, I attended an online speakers conference, Advance Your Reach, on how to tell a story. I had many other things to do that weekend, and I was second-guessing why I had signed up for the event.

I thought back to my Boon of empowering one million moms. I had initially signed up to learn how to improve my speaking skills so I could reach more moms, but when I saw the guest speaker, I smiled at God. This was a divine moment.

Why?

Five years prior to this event, I watched a TED Talk by Catherine (Cat) Hoke, "The Power of Second Chances," and was inspired by her mission.[13] Cat is the founder of three groundbreaking organizations in corrections and rehabilitation, transforming the hustle of America's most overlooked talent pool. She brings incarcerated persons hope and purpose. Many of these people are incarcerated because of their life circumstances or because of what they did when they were suffering from a substance use disorder.

I read her book, *A Second Chance: For You, for Me, and for the Rest of Us,* five years ago and immediately knew I wanted to work with her. I sent her an email but never heard back from her. Seeing her name listed as the guest speaker for this workshop instantly inspired me to try again to connect with her.

At the end of her talk, she shared her email address, and I recognized the door God had opened for me to walk through. It was a divine invitation and not a *coincidence*. A God-wink. He was saying, *You need to reach out to her.*

I knew what I had to do.

The next day, I created a two-minute video introducing myself and sharing how she had inspired me. I also went to her website and researched her new program, Hustle 2.0, a self-directed, in-cell study program for incarcerated people, and sponsored an incarcerated woman who didn't have the means to purchase the program for herself but had the desire to learn.[14]

Several weeks later, Cat responded to my email and sent me an endorsement for this book. The book endorsement is important but not as important as building a relationship with someone who shares similar passions. Not only do we care about incarcerated persons, but we also share interests in quilting, sewing, watercolor art, and oil painting. We agreed to have a Zoom painting session in the future. I'm excited to continue a friendship with Cat and look forward to learning and growing from her influence and experiences.

Connecting with Cat has already expanded my reach and is helping me achieve my Boon, and our relationship will likewise help her achieve her Boon. How will my influence help her? In partnering with her Hustle 2.0 launch, I am asking moms to sponsor inmates. I'll use my platform to spread the word about her program.

Do I know where this friendship will take me? No, but because I recognize this as a divine invitation, and not a hack, I trust that God knows what comes next. My job is to stay focused on my Boon and trust that He will continue to open the right doors.

What Does This Story Have to Do with Hope?

God has a plan for everyone. If we pay attention, we will recognize which parts in our journey are Spirit-led versus havoc-led. When we're focused on the havoc, we don't see God in our lives, and we lose faith. But when we notice His work in our lives, we're able to replace havoc with hope.

In the Havoc

Moms ask me, "What should I do?"

"What have you already tried?" I ask.

"I've helped and helped, but nothing changes."

"What haven't you tried? Maybe you need to look there. Try something new."

"I'm afraid he will die."

"He could die anyway. You can't control his life. What about you? Are you living or slowly dying with your child?"

This last question, *Are you slowly dying with your child,* often causes moms to pause. Does it make you think? I want you to live a full life. God wants you to live fully.

Thanks to our private Facebook group, Moms Letting Go, I've discovered when moms read others' stories, they find hope. They no longer feel alone. Telling our stories gives others hope and helps you heal. We understand parts of your story involve your loved ones, so you don't share everything to keep from shaming them. But you can tell your story without telling their story.

As we said on Day One, telling your story is a part of the healing. Once you do that, you can create our recovery Boon. When you start dreaming of putting purpose to your pain, you will start envisioning what you can do. Once you pray for God to lead you, doors will open. You won't want to walk through some of those doors, but you get to choose.

Once you start dreaming of a different life, you will see it. Everything is created twice. First in your mind. Then in reality.

This is sacred work, your first creation. Don't aim for perfection; take imperfect action. If your *creation* seems fuzzy, don't fret. Time will bring it into focus and allow you to visualize your Boon more clearly.

What is something on your bucket list you haven't prioritized because of your addicted loved one's problem? What is your dream?

If you accomplish this new lifestyle, what will you work toward? What will be the sign you've arrived at this peaceful place? What will this free you to do?

Will you recognize when a Cat Hoke comes into your life?

CLOSE YOUR GAP DAY 10: CREATE YOUR BOON ROAD MAP

It's your turn to create a Boon Sheet. Don't overthink it. Don't aim for perfection. Action is the goal. You won't have clarity yet. You might not even know your Boon but complete the sheet to the best of your ability.

When I first started my mission to help moms, I didn't have a Boon or a Boon Sheet. I just knew I had to find purpose in my pain. My goal was to serve moms and help them navigate through the chaos, the havoc.

Now, every step I take in my coaching, podcasting, and speaking role, I gain more clarity. You will too.

For today's assignment, create your road map by completing a Boon Sheet. This sheet will help you define and articulate your unhackable idea.

Keep in mind no one else can create your Boon, and it can't be contingent upon your addicted loved one's recovery, nor can your Boon be you controlling someone else's actions. Your goals and joy must be independent from other people's actions. Will this be tough? Yes. And you will never attain it if you create a Boon only your children can control. I want you to create a Boon you can achieve.

BOON SHEET   Date: _____

1. **WHO** does my Boon involve?
2. **WHAT** is my Boon?
3. **WHEN** will my Boon be experienced?
4. **WHERE** will my Boon be experienced?
5. **WHY** must I reach this Boon?
6. **HOW** will I begin reaching my Boon (the very first action only)?

Your Signature: _____

Example: Michelle's Boon Sheet

WHO: One million Moms of Addicted Loved Ones
WHAT: To empower moms to embrace self-recovery
WHEN: I want this to happen by 2025.
WHERE: Across the globe. But the Boon party will be at a conference with moms sharing their recovery stories.
WHY: God is counting on me to bring purpose to the pain that addiction has caused my family. With over 270 people dying each day from overdoses, the best people to fight the addiction epidemic are hurting moms. But first they must get well. When moms fight for their children, they can get vocal, intentional, and passionate. But when moms are stuck in the chaos, they don't have the energy or power to fight. That's why my goal is to empower them and help them find purpose in their pain so they have the tools and the hope to fight. Some days, I'm sad and exhausted for moms, but the

reason I do what I do powers me through my day. There is a greater purpose.

HOW: A few of the very first steps I took toward achieving my Boon were starting my podcast, *Moms Letting Go Without Giving Up,* writing the book, and creating a safe Facebook group for moms to gather.

> You don't have to love what you do—if you love why you're doing it.
> **—Tony Colson**

From the All-Mighty Mom Tribe

Brooke's Boon Sheet

WHO: Persons with a criminal or substance disuse history who need transitional housing when they're released from jails or rehabilitation centers

WHAT: Fill the role as secretary for PIVOT TN, Purpose in Valuing Others Today, a housing project for persons who need housing support

WHERE: Maryville, TN, my community

WHEN: As long as it takes to acquire land and build; projected completion date of 2023

WHY: I've seen my son struggle with finding housing options, so I understand and want to be a part of the solution that brings people hope.

HOW: To serve as secretary and a thought-leader

***

Lily's Boon Sheet

WHO: Moms in the All-Mighty Mom Tribe

WHAT: Lead CRAFT (Community Reinforcement and Family Training) recovery education so moms learn how to cope and listen better; practice empathy listening with moms so they build better relationships with their loved ones

WHEN: Starting in January 2022

WHERE: Zoom calls in the All-Mighty Mom Tribe

WHY: I want to serve and share what I've learned through the education I've gained from Dr. Robert J. Meyers because having a son with an SUD helps me understand how important connection is to their recovery.

HOW: By taking the courses and building on my education, I'll be able to gift others with my teaching skills using PowerPoint presentations and coaching methods.

***

Sandy's Boon

My Boon is to find peace; for me, that means spending time enjoying God's creations. I will intentionally rest and find time to enjoy nature, traveling to new places, hiking, kayaking, and sitting to enjoy God's gifts. I will explore, learning interesting cultural and historical information and enjoying local culture and food. I will meditate on God's goodness and promises and practice gratitude. I must do this Boon to experience the peace that only God can provide.

***

Lucretia

WHO: My Boon involves me and moms who need hope on their journey for themselves and their addicted loved ones.

WHAT: To inspire moms to take the steps in their self-care and move forward so they can help others

WHEN: 5,000 Moms by 2025

WHERE: Moms everywhere as they work through and grow in their healing steps. I would love to be involved in a conference, workshop venue, or retreat.

WHY: To teach others what God has shown me through my own personal journey of self-care and learning to communicate with my son during his substance use disorder. I want to encourage, share my passion, and inspire moms to take the next right steps in this difficult season. When moms take care of themselves, change and hope happen. Then they can help others. Hope has a ripple effect.

HOW: I will reach my Boon by working with the All-Mighty Moms and Moms Letting Go groups, facilitating online Bible studies, speaking, and coaching as God leads. I will pray for

God to open new doors of opportunity for me to inspire, encourage, and give hope to moms. Everyone has value, and this life is worth living to the glory of God!

Dissect a Hope Hero

Consult not your fears but your hopes and dreams. Think not about your frustrations, but about your unfulfilled potential. Concern yourself not with what you tried and failed in, but with what is still possible for you to do.

—Pope John XXIII

On June 8, 2021, Jane Marczewski auditioned on *America's Got Talent*. Thirty-years-old, the extremely thin but poised and confident singer and songwriter sang an original song titled "It's Okay," the song that told the story of her past year and her response to the cancer raging in her body. When people asked how she was doing, she explained that she had some cancer in her lungs, spine, and liver but that she was okay. "The doctors only give me a 2 percent chance of living," she said. "But 2 percent isn't 0 percent. Two percent is something."[15]

With the final note of the song, the audience exploded in applause. Simon Cowell had tears in his eyes. He stood, reached for the golden buzzer, and pressed it with zest. Jane was going straight to the live shows. (The judges only press the golden buzzer when an act emotionally moves them.)

Even though doctors gave Jane a miniscule chance of survival, she chose to focus on the positive. Her story told through song resonated with Cowell and the rest of the audience that day because she breathed hope with every note.

Jane is an example of a hope hero. She adopted the name Nightbirde because of three similar dreams she had six months prior to her cancer diagnosis. The dreams came on different nights, and in all of them, birds sang in the trees like they do at dawn. In each dream, however, the skies were dark. Dawn wasn't in sight yet. After these dreams, God spoke to her saying, "You will sing in the dark, even though you have no promise that dawn will come. You will sing in celebration for the thing that isn't here yet."

The quotes below from Nightbirde illustrate the types of stories we want to seek when we feel hopeless.

- "It's important for people to know that I'm so much more than the bad things that have happened to me."
- "You can't wait until life isn't hard anymore until you decide to be happy."
- "Two percent chance of survival is not zero."
- "Just because someone leaves you doesn't mean that love isn't real."
- "It's easy to put your identity in one thing."
- "Some people can't see God because they won't look low enough."
- "There are a lot of people who want to hope for something in their life but are afraid to."[16]

Let's Dissect Nightbirde's Hope

"It's important for people to know that I'm so much more than the bad things that have happened to me." Nightbirde validated her story and who she is. It's important for all of us to share our stories without inhibitions. There's more to you and to your addicted loved one than the bad things that have happened to you both. If you aren't vocal about your story and gifts, they can't find their way into the world to bring others hope.

"You can't wait until life isn't hard anymore until you decide to be happy." Hope is a choice. We will all fight adversity in our lives, but it's how we cope with the stress that makes a difference. Nightbirde has a relationship with God, so when He speaks to her, she can discern that it's His voice. This doesn't just happen. It takes intentionality and a commitment to spend necessary time with ourselves and our high power.

"Two percent chance of survival is not zero." She chooses to focus on the positive —the 2 percent instead of the 98 percent. We can choose to see our loved ones in the grave, or we can choose to see them in recovery.

"Just because someone leaves you doesn't mean that love isn't real." Think about this in relation to your situation. For many of us, our children have *left* us. Maybe not in the physical sense but in the emotional and spiritual sense. The enemy has hacked them. We grieve for who they used to be and the love they used to share in their relationship with us. It's important to remember our children love us, even though we might not feel it or see it. The enemy has your child in hiding, but as long as your children are living, there is hope you will feel their love again.

"It's easy to put your identity in one thing." Motherhood can steal a mom's identity. When we spend our lives making our children a priority and can't find our own sense of self, we're risking happiness. Why? Because we can't control our adult children—what they do, who they hang with, and how they live their lives. Sometimes it's easier to *only* be someone's mom and nothing more, but it's not a fulfilling life.

"Some people can't see God because they won't look low enough." Consider these thoughts from Nightbirde's blog as you look for God:

I spent three months propped against the wall. On nights that I could not sleep, I laid in the tub like an insect, staring at my reflection in the shower knob. I vomited until I was hollow. I rolled up under my robe on the tile. The bathroom floor became my place to hide, where I could scream and be ugly; where I could sob and spit and eventually doze off, happy to be asleep, even with my head on the toilet.

Even on days when I'm not so sick, sometimes I go lay on the mat in the afternoon light to listen for Him. I know it sounds crazy, and I can't really explain it, but God is in there—even now. I have heard it said that some people can't see God because they won't look low enough, and it's true.

If you can't see him, look lower. God is on the bathroom floor.[17]

"There are a lot of people who want to hope for something in their life but are afraid to." They're afraid of being let down. Maybe they've hoped repeatedly for something, and their dreams didn't come true, so they gave up on hope. Hope is what we need more than anything, no matter what situation we're facing. Don't be afraid to hope. Hopelessness can be a sign of depression and/or learned helplessness. Both

are important to understand because we need hope to help us cope. If you feel like you no longer have hope, please reach out to your physician or a therapist. Don't be afraid to hope.

CLOSE YOUR GAP DAY 11: DISSECT YOUR HOPE

For today's assignment, answer these questions:

- When you envision hope, what do you see?
- Make a list. Share it with someone.
- Which of Nightbirde's quotes inspire you the most and why?
- What part of your hope outcome can you control?

Notes from the All-Mighty Mom Tribe

Brooke

My Hope Vision:

- To be seen, known, and accepted is the deep desire of my heart
- To see, know, and accept others is my greatest aspiration

A wish I have is to be connected to a group of people. I want a place to belong, where others are willing to listen and hold space. I want to be valued for who I am, even when my way of being is different from the norm. I want some place to enter and know someone cares and will not judge.

I never had the privilege of receiving approval or affirmation in a family, so I crave these things in the depths of my soul. As the new year begins, this is an intention I am putting into the universe.

What part can I control?

- Learn language that helps others understand my feelings
- Choose to enter groups that have the potential to be safe spaces
- Make intentional attempts to trust that others can be generous in their thoughts and actions
- Try, try, and try again without taking the end result as rejection. At this age, there will be many challenges to belonging.

***

Lily

I can relate to several of Nightbirde's quotes.

I do feel grief that my son has left me. He is not emotionally available anymore. He hasn't been for a while. He used to be my buddy. We would go to movies together, meet for lunch on my day's off, and just spend quiet afternoons together. That hasn't happened in years. I miss him.

"Two percent chance of survival is not zero" reminds me of my mother and her strong belief that God would be her healer. She believed His reports, not those of the medical community, when she had cancer. Throughout her treatment, she believed she would be cured, and she was.

Hope is my belief that something will change, that something will happen. I pray for a certain outcome; however, I can never be sure that it will happen. I believe that God cares about our lives and knows the desires of our hearts. But we can't control what other people will do with their free will.

DAY 12

Discover Your Hope

*Informed optimism doesn't mean you only look at the
bright side. It means you don't overlook the bright side. If
you won't see possibility, you can't solve problems. If you
can't imagine a best case, you don't make things better. The
greatest antidote to fear is grounded hope*

—Adam Grant

What is hope?

The word *hope* occurs in the NLT Bible 159 times,
the KJV 133 times, and the NIV version 175 times. It's an
important word.

Hope is anticipating that something you desire will come
true. It's wanting something so badly the anticipation of it
keeps you excited for the future. It's an optimistic state of
mind, a positive outcome. Hope can make a tough situation
bearable. Hope helps us define and visualize what we want
for our future. Hope can provide the key to making our lives
better.

God wants us to have hope. He gives this gift to us by promising to be with us in the difficult times. He doesn't take away our pain but helps us cope with our pain—if we let Him.

Hope is listening to a recovering addict's story, a light in a dark alley, the calming winds after a hurricane. It's the promise of a better tomorrow.

Since we know hope is important, shouldn't we search for it? Yes! Yet so many moms give up.

I asked moms in the private Facebook group, Moms Letting Go, how they felt about and understood hope. Here are some of their answers to the question, *What is hope?*

- Useless.
- Something I'm tired of trying to have.
- Something that brings me up when I'm down. I believe in prayer, so I'm waiting for my Savior's time. I am impatient, but I know my prayer will be answered. I believe I will get my son back.
- What is found when you put your trust and understanding in God's hands and leave it there.
- Faith that God loves me and is always with me.
- Eternal.
- What keeps me going.
- Sometimes fleeting.
- Possible where there is life.
- Something to hang onto regardless of what the circumstances look like.
- Not giving up.
- Jesus.

You can see that hope means different things to different people. Hope isn't about ignoring your pain. It's acknowledging the pain and trusting God for a better future.

Hope is powerful. Mentally, hope gives you the strength to go from one day to the next. Physically, it causes your brain to release endorphins which creates a similar effect as morphine.[18] Spiritually, it does not disappoint (Romans 5:5).

Hope is your ally. Hold onto it with all your might.

> *I believe hope is as vital to the brain as the oxygen we breathe.*
> **—Terry Small**

When we feel hopeless, it's important to look for ways to hope again instead of staying stuck.

Ways to Find or Recapture Hope

- Believe that you have some control over the outcome and take action to that end.

- Learn how to strengthen our faith.

- If you're angry at yourself or someone else, forgive. Forgiveness will allow you to break free from long-held grudges that might be keeping you in hopelessness.

- Look for what you want to find. Seek out positive people, humorous moments, and transformational stories.

- Connect with others who understand.

- Avoid comparisons.

- Find hope heroes—those role models who have overcome adversity. Allow them to show you the way.

- Listen to stories of the people who have recovered.

- Focus on things you can control.

- Start a project you've always wanted to try.

- Get involved in the solution.

- Believe you can achieve your goals.
- Tap into past resiliencies. I lead workshops in the jail where incarcerated people share stories of when they've been strong in their lives.
- Perform a random act of kindness.
- Make your mess a message for others by speaking to support groups.
- Chase your dreams. Establishing your Boon helps.
- Do something small every day toward finding hope so it becomes a new habit.
- Practice prayer or meditation. Do it alone and with others. We see a new perspective when we pray with someone else. We're able to borrow hope from them.
- Take comfort in not knowing the outcome or being responsible for it. Just as much as X might happen, X might not happen.
- Start a gratitude journal.

Hope is a shared human experience. When we express our hopes with others and surround ourselves with hope builders, we see hope and feel positive energy. Hope emerges through interactions with the people who surround us.

In 2008, Duane Bidwell and his colleague Dr. Donald Batisky, a pediatric nephrologist at Emory University School of Medicine in Atlanta, analyzed data from a diverse group of children suffering from end-stage renal failure. The researchers identified five main pathways to hope:

1. *Maintaining identity by continuing to participate in activities and relationships that help people retain a sense of self outside diagnosis and treatment.*

2. *Finding community through formal and informal connections. Community helped the children and their families understand they were not alone in living with this disease. Community forms through conversation, visitation, consultation, and participation in daily activities.*

3. *Claiming power by taking an active role in treatment by setting goals, self-advocating, monitoring, and maintaining one's health.*

4. *Attending to spirituality, activated through religious, spiritual, and other contemplative practices.*

5. *Developing wisdom, which involves both gaining pragmatic, medical wisdom derived from one's own experience and finding ways to "give back."*[19]

What Can You Apply from These Findings?

1. Be authentic to yourself, your values, and your dreams despite your plight as the mom of an addicted loved one.

2. Find a community so you don't feel alone. Many other moms are trying to cope with the same problems you face daily. Get involved in a community by sharing your emotions, affirming others, and staying active.

3. Stay connected to your higher power in a way that helps boost your spirituality.

4. Study addiction and share what you have learned from your experiences with others who need to hear your wisdom.

Don't Stay in Hopelessness too Long

If you've ever hung out with someone who is hopeless, you might have tried unsuccessfully to bring them hope. You may have eventually abandoned the friendship because their lack of energy depleted yours.

Hopelessness is the belief that nothing will ever change. When we're hopeless, we're resistant to change. We don't want to try anything new because we don't think our wish will come true.

If we stay in this place for a brief time, just long enough to acknowledge our feelings and identify them, we can grieve. We can grieve for the loss of hope. Ignoring the grief invites it to fester beneath the surface. It builds until it rises to the surface like an angry boil when we least expect it. We won't heal by ignoring grief.

It is important to acknowledge feelings of hopelessness. We can journal about it, cover it with a soothing balm like a prayer, worship music, or tears, and then stand and move on. Sometimes it's necessary to share our feelings with a friend before we can move on. When we share our hopelessness with others, we release the energy. We let it go. The energy is released into the air, and if we're among hope builders who listen to and validate us, they will show us the positives we may have missed. Eventually, time, healing, and attention restore our hope.

The Hope Cycle

Observe the diagram below.

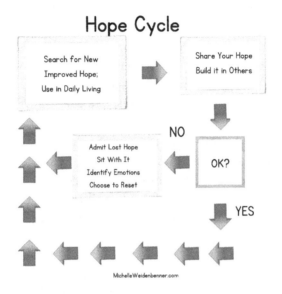

Hope is a continuous cycle. It requires ongoing renewal.

Step One: Search for new, improved ways to find hope. (Refer to the list earlier in this chapter for suggestions.)

Step Two: Share hope with others. Hope is a social resource. You find and embrace it through interactions with the people your surround yourself with. Share your hope with others in a safe community, one that understands you, affirms your journey, and doesn't judge you. Surrounding yourself with hope builders is important. Identify who they are in your life. If you don't have enough of them, search for more.

When your friends lose hope, help build it in them. When we strengthen hope in others, it strengthens our resiliency.

Step Three: If you lose hope along the way, stop and assess what has changed. Allow yourself to sit with hopelessness but not for too long. Have a pity party and grieve for your loss. What emotions are you feeling? How can you reset and begin to look for hope again? Make a choice to renew your hope. Look for those hope builders you identified and intentionally reach out to them. Ask them to help you rediscover hope. Be specific about your needs so they know how to help you.

Begin Again: Look for new ways to find hope. If you need to research your options for a while, take the time to work thorough solutions before you start again.

> *When moms recover, they become hope builders for others.*

Learned Helplessness Can Cause Hopelessness

Learned helplessness occurs when a person suffers from a sense of powerlessness and the feeling that they will fail before they even try. Learned helplessness can steal hope.

When my son was in grade school, I thought he had a learning disability, but a counselor said it was learned helplessness. I hadn't heard of this concept before, so I researched it.

Our addicted loved ones often feel helpless when they try to recover and fail repeatedly. They think they'll fail again, so they think, *What's the point of trying?*

It's important for moms to understand this condition and to know that learned helplessness is behavior that can be unlearned. By sharing ways to find or renew hope, we can empower and encourage our loved ones. We can be their hope builders and equip them to overcome learned helplessness.

Way Power versus Will Power

We can want to find hope but not know the way. If we see a way forward, we're more likely to develop the will to make it happen. We need both—the way and the will.

Regarding your Boon, think of a way to develop both the will power and the way power to tackle your challenge. What do you need to do to move forward?

CLOSE YOUR GAP DAY 12: DISCOVER YOUR HOPE

For today's assignment, consider the following:

- Using the ways to find and recapture hope examples above, list four ways you will look for hope to achieve your dreams or Boon.
- Observe the hope cycle. Where are you today in the cycle regarding achieving your Boon?
- Nelson Mandela risked his life to serve others. He brought people hope when they had none. Identify a Hope Hero, like Mandela, to study for inspiration. Journal why you chose your hero and what you learned from him or her.

Notes from the All-Mighty Mom Tribe

Sandy

I look for hope to achieve my dreams/Boon in the following four ways:

1. I continue to read scripture, read and hear other's thoughts about faith, attend church and small groups, and talk with other Christians to grow my faith.
2. I am an active member in the All-Mighty Mom Tribe. This allows me to connect and grow stronger with other moms who truly understand what I am going through.
3. I have learned what I can and cannot control. I focus on those things I can control and turn those things I cannot control over to God.
4. I try to encourage others every day. I enjoy creating gifts for others.

In looking at the Hope Cycle, I have been through all eight stages. I am currently in stage four and feel hopeful.

***

Lucretia

I will look for hope to achieve my Boon in these four ways:

1. Ask and seek God for direction, clarity, and wisdom.
2. Ask prayer partners and truth tellers to diligently pray with me about my Boon.
3. Take steps that will empower me to learn.
4. Take classes or courses to grow.

In the Hope Cycle, I'm researching a solution to my problem so I can find hope in accomplishing my Boon.

Hope Hero—I have always liked Zig Ziglar and his positive attitude about everything. His most famous quote is this: "You can have everything in life you want if you will just help enough other people get what they want." It comes from Ziglar's book Great Quotes from Zig Ziglar: 250 Inspiring Quotes from the Master Motivator and Friends.

PART THREE

Deliberate Mom Focus

DAY 13

Urgency: Create Your Space

Deadlines refine the mind. They remove variables like exotic materials and processes that take too long. The closer the deadline, the more likely you'll start thinking way outside the box.

—Adam Savage

I n Part Two, we focused on the anatomy of hope. In this part, you'll discover how to attain a Deliberate Mom Focus using Focus Filter #1, urgency.

I can't stress it enough: before you can expect your addicted loved one to change, you must focus on how you can change. Addiction is a family disease; everybody plays a part. Often moms need to play a new and different part.

Every day in our private Facebook group, moms ask questions about their addicted children and how best to help them. Let me share one such question:

My daughter is pregnant and wants to keep her child, but she wants to live with me. She is actively using and smoking cigarettes. I worry about the effects of these substances on her unborn child. I am not able to care for her and her child. I don't know what to do. I feel terrible about putting her on the street when she is carrying a child.

What advice would you give?

It's easy to see solutions when we're not emotionally attached. But once we're involved in the enabling cycle, it's tough to stop. Moms feel a need to fix their loved one's problems. We think fixing or eliminating the consequences of our child's actions shows we care.

True caring is holding your child's hand and praying with her and for her, expressing empathy for her difficult plight while empowering her to take responsibility for her life and the consequences that arise from her choices. Caring says, "You can do this," when we'd rather tell her, "This would be easier without your addiction." We don't say this because, until she's willing to admit she has a problem, she will deny she uses substances—even if it's blatant to us.

If we lecture, shame, and *should* our child, the conversation can escalate into a heated battle. People who use know how to manipulate us. The best thing to do is master the art of listening and staying calm.

Caring also means having a healthy boundary plan for our self-care and not allowing guilt to disrupt the plan. I recommend moms sit with their spouses or significant others and discuss their boundaries. They need to show their addicted adult child a strong united front. Your child might not like that you're setting new boundaries together, but it will help her see you're serious.

What to Do

The most effective boundaries begin with a list of your expectations. If you're working with a family therapist, let this person help you and your spouse build your recovery plan.

Then you and your spouse should set a date for each expectation. For example, one boundary item might look like this: you need to move out by _____. Write down the deadline. Finally, you need agree on how you will enforce each boundary. What consequences will she face if she doesn't abide by your new rule? List that too.

Next, meet with your addicted loved one when she is not under the influence and explain that things are going to change. Tell your adult child that you're working on *your* recovery plan. Show her your plan. Sign it while she's watching. Ask her to sign it too. If she chooses not to, don't press it. Leave the list of boundaries in a place where she can see it and let her know you will enforce it whether she agrees to it or not.

Like a two-year-old child, she might kick and scream and hate you for doing what you need to do. She won't understand. If she's under the influence of a substance, she is operating with upside-down logic. She might feel anxiety or be triggered to use. Allow her to own her feelings and cope with them her way. You are not responsible for her rage. If you believe your life is in danger, calmly leave your home.

Many will choose to skip the deadlines, but these dates define your urgency. They help your ALO understand the seriousness of your list. Creating urgency gives you focus and a powerful tool. Every day matters.

Let's look at the troubled grandmother scenario again. In this case, an innocent child's life is at stake. Who will care for the baby after she's born? It complicates the problem.

If we let it play out and allow our child to accept the consequences, we can see a variety of scenarios. The good thing is this is not our decision. She gets to choose. In fact, it may help you to use that as a mantra. Keep telling yourself, "My child gets to choose. My child gets to choose."

The Possibilities

Looking at the possibilities can be tough. She could end up on the streets and continue using. Depending on which substances she uses, the baby could be born with an addiction or suffer from other health issues. If the baby is born with an addiction, your daughter could lose her parenting rights. The baby could be placed in a foster home.

Guilt might try to convince you to do something to avoid this scenario. But your boundaries and deadlines will help you practice self-care first.

Yes, you can still meet with your daughter to listen and pray. Help her take responsibility with questions: *What will you do? What are your options?* Affirm her with encouraging responses. *It sounds like you're in a difficult spot. It doesn't seem like you have any good choices, but which will be the easiest for you right now?*

Guiding her to make her own choices is wicked tough. You might not agree with her decisions, and you might be tempted to interject your opinion, but this is where you must honor her boundaries. She won't grow up or stop using if you make the decisions for her.

You might say, "What will my friends and family say about me abandoning my child and unborn grandchild?" Everybody has an opinion, and you will probably hear what they think. Let them know you love your daughter, and you're not abandoning her. Show them you're setting healthy boundaries. Explain that you and your spouse agreed on this action plan because you are in recovery and learning healthy ways to handle these situations. Be the boss of you and stand tough in your decisions.

On the other hand, your daughter could go to a homeless shelter, get sober, find a job, take parenting classes, and continue with a recovery plan. She will still have problems, and you'll be tempted to help if you see her really trying. Above all, honor your boundaries and don't fix anything. You can be there emotionally. Hold her hand and listen without interjecting your opinion. (Your tongue will bleed, but this is necessary for her forward progress). Acknowledge each of her decisions, even if you disagree with them. Watch for and mention her forward progress. Congratulate her on the things she's doing to improve her life.

Worst Case Scenario for You and Your Boon

Allowing your daughter to stay with you, caring for her, and micromanaging her actions will fill your life with chaos. Your focus will be on her instead of you. You'll be the police, monitoring her support meeting attendance. You'll give her a curfew, and you'll have to follow through with the consequences if she doesn't abide. She will treat you with disrespect, and your overall health will suffer.

When we remove the consequences of our loved one's actions, they don't grow up or learn from their mistakes. The pleasure of using outweighs the pain. If we allow them to accept the consequences of their behavior, then they will struggle with the pain and hopefully be motivated to change.

When we take responsibility for our loved ones, we inadvertently tell them they can't do it, we don't believe in their ability, and we can do it better—whatever *it* is. Maybe we can do some things better, but if we want them to change and take responsibility, they need to believe in themselves, that they can do life on their own.

When we focus on the urgency of our situation, it helps us set healthy boundaries and establish a deadline. Additionally, our boundaries and deadlines will create a sense of urgency for our loved one.

One More Deadline

Having a deadline for your Boon is important too. Just because you have a destination doesn't mean you have a motivation. The thing that will get you moving in full force is urgency, your Focus Filter #1.

Urgency is baked into a deadline. What will it cost if you don't reach your goal by the date you envision? Goals without deadlines are pipe dreams. There needs to be something at stake. A penalty will create that motivation.

Urgency is the first way to create magnetic focus to accomplish your dream. The urgency for my Boon begins with my age. I'm sixty-four years old. I have a lot to do in my life, and my days are running out. If I'm going to impact one million moms of addicted loved ones, I must work faster.

When we discussed this book's deadline, we decided it would launch on Mother's Day, 2022. This means we need to complete the book at least six months ahead of time so we can complete the editing process, load book information to the selling sites, buy our ISBN numbers, design the book cover, and write a press release.

What is my penalty for not completing this book in time to launch on Mother's Day? I will lose the traction I could have gained with a Mother's Day launch. Mother's Day fits the theme of this book, and losing that will impact lives.

CLOSE YOUR GAP DAY 13: CREATE YOUR SPACE

Choosing a deadline for your boundaries is important because if you don't, you'll go in circles and never climb out of the addiction chaos tornado.

You have two challenges for today:

1. First build your list of boundaries and deadlines for your addicted loved one.
2. Next, choose the deadline for attaining your Boon. Include your motivation. What is your urgency? What will the penalty be if you're not done by this date?

Many people have anxiety due to the number of distractions in our lives. When you add the drama and chaos created by our loved one, the distractions multiply. If we're not careful, these interruptions become addictions. Every time we're distracted, it creates dopamine loops. These distractions cause us to watch for messages from our addicted loved one. The more we look, the more we feel we must look. Some moms sleep with their phones nearby, so they don't miss the notifications in the middle of the night. They can't stop this obsessive habit. They can't turn their phones off. They can't turn their anxiety off.

Imagine having the ability to burn through any obstacle or distraction. Having a deadline with urgency and a penalty will significantly increase your outcome and enable you to move steadily forward on the path toward your Boon.

Notes from the All-Mighty Mom Tribe
Brooke

By February 2022, I will have a career that is fulfilling and flexible enough to meet my family's needs. I will focus on myself and the path to becoming a productive wage earner, and I will allow my addicted loved one to make his own decisions. I want the dignity of feeling accomplished in a career, and I give my loved one permission to be where he feels most gratified.

***

Lucretia

Three years ago, I knew I had to make major changes. I couldn't continue to live in an emotional state all the time. My husband and I created a plan to move forward. We had to take ownership of what enabling was doing to us and to our son. I gave our son his move out date and steps to work toward that. He did nothing. He didn't think I was serious about selling the house and moving.

At that time, he, his baby's momma, and the baby were living with us. We thought we could help them get back on their feet. It cost us more than I want to admit. We told them their time was up, and they had to leave.

Emotions ran high, angry words flew, and police were called. We kept the baby. Afterward I breathed, walked, took yoga, went to the chiropractor, and got massages to start my recovery. I had three big garage sales and sold all kinds of things on Facebook marketplace. Then, during COVID-19 this last year, our house sold. We downsized and moved. It felt so good! I know this was a major step, but I had to be in a different physical place, a new place to start over for my recovery. I even gave my two little dogs back to their original owners. I loved my dogs but didn't need or want anything else to take care of. The focus was my self-care.

DAY 14

Agency: Choose Your Inputs

What takes up space in your thoughts can control your life.

B ecoming an Unhackable Mom of an Addicted Loved One is impossible unless you recognize your own space. In the last chapter, I introduced our first Focus Filter, urgency, and you owned what your space looks like. Your boundaries and deadlines may need to be adjusted as you move forward, but for now, you are working toward a goal. Once you have something as important as your Boon to focus on, you can heal.

Today, I've asked Crystal Waltman, recovering addict, Unhackable Coach, and author of *Quitting to Win,* to lend her expertise to our second Focus Filter, agency.

***

Addiction comes in many forms. The trigger reveals your agency. Agency is built by everything that is consumed through the five senses. They offer input ports for those things that will bring peace or a trigger. What you hear, watch, listen to, and consume—in any form—can or will make or break you.

Those of us born with the addiction gene must make a daily choice to turn the addiction on or off by what we put into our bodies. Agency is everything! Your capacity to act independently and make better choices can be grown, cleaned up, uncluttered, and eventually made unhackable.

Addiction is a mental illness, making agency the most important factor. For many years in my addiction, if I was happy, I would drink. If I was sad, I would drink, Whenever I felt uncomfortable, I would drink. Instead of taking inventory of my agency, I reached for anything numbing.

As a mother and sober athlete, having gone through an inventory of my life and making amends several times, I've had to build my agency. I use a childlike phrase to keep it simple— garbage in, garbage out. Originally a computer term, GIGO applies to our senses too. What we input determines our agency.

***

When not working, I play pickleball. It's the fastest growing sport in America.[20] The game includes keeping the ball in play, using my racket to place it where my opponent can't hit a return, and keeping score. I can't think of anything else when I'm concentrating on the game.

When I'm on the court, I don't worry about my children or grandchildren. I don't worry about paying bills or making dinner. I'm totally absorbed in the game. It's like a game of chess. Every thought involves strategy—ball placement, my opponents' weak points, and the next shot.

After I play, I typically think about what I did well and what I need to improve. After I play, I'm always more focused. I get more done than if I hadn't exercised.

What about you? What helps take you away from your obsessive thoughts? What do you feed your brain during your down time? When we find something we love to do, something that challenges our mind and requires physical concentration, we become much more focused on our work.

I know when I play pickleball I'm going to sweat, so before I go, I fill up a water jug and mix in electrolytes. If I don't, I will be slow, shaky, and have low stamina. What I take in determines what I put out.

What you put in will create you. Every input shapes what you put out.

Adding Healthy Input

A year into my son's recovery, we took our grandchildren to visit him and his wife. They brought their lunches in bags and had scraped together enough to take their kids for ice cream. Both had full-time jobs, and they were doing so many things right, but financial progress was slow.

"Can I make a suggestion?" I asked. (Up until this time, I had always interjected my opinion without asking permission.)

"Sure," he said.

"Dad and I feel like you're losing hope. You've been doing well for a year now, but your sober-living arrangement and having to pay $1,500 a month for rent is difficult, to say the least. We're proud of you, but you need encouragement. Something more. Would you consider working with a coach?"

"A coach?"

"Yes, not necessarily a recovery coach, but a life coach. Someone who can build you up and show you how to rear-range your life for success."

He didn't hesitate long. "That sounds great."

Years prior, I had learned the value of having a personal coach, someone who would speak truth, push me, and bring my fears to the surface so I could accomplish more. I had worked with Trudy Menke, a John Maxwell Coach, who helped me become a greater version of myself. (I'm still a work in progress.) I knew the value of what a great coach could do.

After interviewing several people, I found Jesse Harless, the author of *If Not You, Then Who?* Jesse is a leader in the addiction recovery and mental health space. His passion is to help individuals and purpose-driven organizations share their voices to co-create a better world. He met with Ryan to see if they were a good fit, and they were. I was excited to give Ryan this gift of coaching. I could finally do something to help without trying to fix his problems, and he was receptive. Jesse and Ryan worked together for six months.

> Your environment will become you. Surround yourself with people who have the same dream as you, who have accomplished what you want and more.
> —**Keshia Chanté**

During that time, Ryan received tremendous input. He learned great strategies for coping and how to lead himself to success. He began to believe in himself and found passion and the courage to search for something bigger than anything he had imagined. With Jesse's input, Ryan created daily weekly, and monthly intentions; an annual financial, personal, health, and career goal; and a five-year plan.

Last week, Ryan bought his first big rig semi cab. He has hauled freight before but never with his own truck and his own company. When he shared his news with us, he said, "Jesse planted this idea and helped me dream big."

While Ryan was driving across state lines with his previous job, he chose to listen to the voices of people who could inspire him, motivate him, and teach him about a business that interested him. Once he knew he wanted to own his own truck, he connected with one person who motivated him to pursue his dream and coached him on how to start his business.

Once your Boon is clear, you can also surround yourself with others doing what you want to do and find motivation, inspiration, and a clear path.

***

Crystal asks, "How does one become the master of their own agency? By keeping it simple. I have five non negotiables for building agency to manage mental health."

> Alcoholism is a thinking problem, not a drinking problem.
> **—Crystal Waltman**

"When I experience the RID triggers—restlessness, irritability, and discontentment—I HALT and do a quick inventory check: am I hungry, angry, lonely or tired?"[21]

The Foundation of Agency: Water, Sleep, Food, Movement, and Connection

- **Water**: Eighty percent of Americans walk around dehydrated. This number one preventable ailment can be self-corrected. Signs of dehydration include fatigue, hunger, brain fog, headaches, body aches, and tight muscles. Each person should be consuming about half their body weight in ounces daily. Add an extra twelve ounces for a workout and eight more for extremely hot days.

- **Sleep**: Develop a good sleep regimen. Start your routine at the same time every night. Shut off all screens an hour before bed. Wear comfortable clothes. Have the room at a pleasant temperature. Review your daily gratitude list, pray by counting them on your fingers. Meditate to relax the nervous system.

- **Food**: Food can be your greatest medicine or the slowest form of poison. Eat God-made food; if it comes in a package, there is probably a better choice. For more food tips, go to crystalwaltman.com.

- **Movement**: Your body is made of systems with the brain as its supercomputer. Help yourself out by moving every day. Keep it simple and sustainable. Thirty minutes or 7,000 steps is a great goal.

- **Connection**: Both with friends and God. The opposite of addiction is connection. Stay connected with the ones who fill your cup as well as your higher power.

Tip—It's easy to combine movement and connection. When a friend calls and asks me for lunch, I say, "Yes. I would love to meet for a quick juice and a long walk and talk." This way I get movement and fresh air, plus people are more likely to let their emotions out when they are moving and being interrupted by a restaurant server.

Once you have urgency in place (Day 13), your inputs will become easier to clarify, and one day they will bring you joy. Anything that doesn't align with your values has no place giving you input.

CLOSE YOUR GAP DAY 14: AGENCY: CHOOSE YOUR INPUTS

What will you allow into your mind, body, and spirit? Are the things you're absorbing helping you achieve your Boon? What can you eliminate? What can you add? Where do you want to grow? Does what you eat help feed your idea? Do the nutrients you ingest give you energy?

For today, keep it simple. Think about all your inputs: your smart phone, radio, podcast, TV, friends, family, books, magazines, and social media feed. Try to remember the last time you let an input become a trigger and gave your peace away. What medium did it come through? If you cannot eliminate that person, voice, or platform, then use the rule of halves. Reduce their input by half. Less is more. Don't complicate things. Remember the three Cs of addiction: you did not *cause* it, you cannot *control* it, you cannot *cure* it.

What can you control? Your hope and your peace.

When I was living in addiction, if my core relationship was not comfortable, I would have a debilitating day and cause havoc to those around me. When I switched and focused on my higher power, I found my peace.

> If someone or something is driving you crazy, stop giving them the keys.
> — **Crystal Waltman**

***

Create a plan to input things that will benefit your Boon and help grow your agency.

Below are a few examples:

- Read or listen to books on addiction. (Thirty minutes a day)

- Listen to spiritual /worship music. (Twenty minutes a day)

- Explore Bible studies or devotionals. (Fifteen minutes each morning)

- Listen to podcasts while working out. (Thirty minutes a week)

- Replace an hour of TV with journaling.

- Attend two weekly support programs. (Like our Tribe)
- Indulge in ten minutes of positive daily affirmations.
- Connect with people accomplishing a similar Boon.
- Talk to someone who can help you achieve your Boon.
- Meet with a recovering addict who has been sober for two years or more.
- Research and follow someone reaching goals like yours.
- Do one thing that makes you uncomfortable every day.

Grab a calendar and a pencil. Set deadlines for your inputs. Review them in thirty days so you can see your progress.

Notes from the All-Mighty Mom Tribe

Sandy

Zig Ziglar was the first motivational speaker I remember hearing as a guidance counselor. He made a huge impression on me. Of his many great, inspiring quotes, one has stuck with me: "Your attitude determines your altitude." We can control our attitude (which can be difficult), and when we do, so many other things begin to change.

***

Brooke

Our family gave up television during the 2016 election, and we've never gone back to the big box trance. I fill the time previously occupied by TV with books, podcasts, and Audible. It's amazing how much more productive my idle time has become! I listen to podcasts while I exercise, clean house, or cook. My mind is constantly being renewed by things that cause my neurons to fire in a positive way. I am grateful for modern technology and the ability to fill my mind with knowledge.

DAY 15

Energy: Allocate Your Attention

Time is the most valuable coin in your life.
You and you alone will determine how that coin will be spent.
Be careful that you do not let other people spend it for you.

—Carl Sandburg

When the alarm goes off, I lay in bed and stretch for two minutes. I think about my day and what's on my calendar. Once I'm out of bed, I head to the bathroom and take my thyroid meds. During that time, I think about what I'm going to wear, who I'm going to see, where I left my glasses, and what I will eat for breakfast and dinner. I make nearly one hundred decisions before I leave my bedroom. Some days, I'm exhausted after being awake for only five minutes.

Moms' pre-work routines include planning and prepping dinner, throwing in a load or two of laundry, watering the plants, and any number of other tasks. We get a lot done in one hour. I used to have a race every morning to see how much I could accomplish before I left for work.

What about you? How many decisions do you make a day? Probably too many to count. In addition to the everyday planning, we make decisions about our addicted loved ones. Moms in our private group beg for prayers and suggestions for their weary thoughts each day. This is one from today:

Once again, I have a scenario I'm not sure how to handle. My addicted daughter recently got out of rehab. She's here with me and her son. They've recommended outpatient rehab to prevent relapse. This is great because we've never had that before. She is looking into sober living. But the only one she can afford is a sober house in the same neighborhood where she used to get her drugs. I want her to stay here and not be stressed about a place to live if she's sober. I know it's going to take a while for her to get on her feet. My husband doesn't want her here. I'm so tired of this. Not sure what I'm going to do. But she feels the tension, so she doesn't really want to be here. I'm so proud of her right now.

Do you hear her anxiety? She thinks her daughter's problems belong to her. Not only is she making decisions for her own life, but she's also trying to make decisions for her adult child. This leads to exhaustion. It's no wonder that, by the end of our day, we say things like:

I am . . .

- spent.
- empty.
- drained.
- stressed.
- maxed.

- dragging.
- depleted.
- overwhelmed.
- hopeless.

In the two previous sections we covered urgency and agency. In this section, we're covering the final Focus Filter— energy. What merits your attention? What if you could allocate your energy and conserve it so you could focus on the most important things and have enough stamina to manage your self-care and hug yourself with compassion?

A Few Tips

If you automate your *insignificant* decisions, you will be able to focus more of your energy on the bigger decisions. Decision fatigue is real, and taking steps to conserve our energy can be a significant step toward unhackability.

> Where attention goes, energy flows and results show.
> —**T. Harv Eker**

Focusing on something we can't control, like our addicted loved ones, zaps our energy, and at the end of the day, we have nothing to show for it except our drained emotional, mental, spiritual, and physical health.

If we want to accomplish great things, we must find a way to guard our energy. If we let people suck the life out of us, we must stop giving them the straw.

Consider automating these tasks:

- Every Sunday, choose your wardrobe for the rest of the week.
- Create a monthly Bible verse calendar.
- Create a monthly dinner calendar. Ask other family members to add their favorites to the list so you aren't the only one responsible. It will help them learn how to contribute.
- Hire someone to clean your home every two weeks.

- Order a meal service twice a week.
- Order groceries online.
- Use Amazon Prime subscription services to automatically re-order the items you routinely use.
- If you have grandchildren living with you, invite them to take on chores. Teach them how to sort their laundry and how to use the washing machine. Empower them by teaching them life skills that will help them later too.
- Choose an exercise routine that works for your body and your schedule. Write it on your calendar and show up like it's a planned meeting.
- Get up at the same time every day.
- Make your bed every day.

A Big Part of Conserving Energy Means Making Every Moment Count

A friend asked me to show her how Spotify works so she could create a playlist for her mother's funeral. We lived in different states, so I couldn't see her in person. I created a video tutorial for her and shared the playlist that I had created for my mother's funeral. I went out of my way to create and email her my homemade video tutorial. She never thanked me or acknowledged that she received my video.

The next time I talked to her, I asked if she had received my instructions. She said she did but hadn't watched the video because she didn't have time. I was frustrated because I have very limited time, just like her. I wished she would have told me that she didn't need my help, but she didn't, and I ended up feeling like I'd wasted my time.

We all have the same amount of time, but we don't always choose to use it constructively. I used my time to do something for my friend that she hadn't asked for. My time and energy would have been better spent writing another chapter or learning something new.

How we use our time determines who we become. If you listen to addiction podcasts or audiobooks while you exercise or drive, you will learn on the go. Not only will the time pass faster, but you will also broaden your knowledge, expand your mindset, and conserve your energy.

***

Crystal Waltman illustrates the potential financial value for each hour of our time:

> When you've set up urgency and your agency is crystal clear, you don't waste time. For instance, look at how much time you spend on social media and phone screen time. Then consider your hourly billable rate. Even if your primary job is homemaker or you volunteer, how much would it cost if they had to pay someone to replace you. Is it $10, $100, $1000, or $10,000 an hour? Let's assume you give your phone or social media one hour each day. Multiply your hourly rate by 365. A consultant who bills $100 on average would have burned $36,500 on social media or phone scrolling. In seventy years, the waste would increase to more than 25,000 hours or 2.5 million dollars.

CLOSE YOUR GAP DAY 15: ENERGY: ALLOCATE YOUR ATTENTION

For today's mission, start small. Rather than automating every decision, choose one. Once you see how powerful automating is, you will want to identify other decisions to automate.

Get those easy ones out of the way so you can focus on what matters most.

In the space below, identify one thing you can pre-decide right now. This step will help you see how easy it is. And you'll be surprised at your increased energy because you will have one less decision to make every day.

You may struggle with some decisions you automate. When I wrote each of my novels, for instance, I made the decision to start writing every weekday at 8:30 a.m. and keep writing until I finished 1,500 words. I stayed faithful to this schedule until I completed the 50,000-word book. Some days I stared at a blank page, but the thought of getting my work done so I could do something fun helped. Plus, the reward of a completed manuscript proved to be great motivation.

Decisions You Can Pre-Plan Regarding Your Addicted Loved One

In addition to your productivity automations, you can automate your boundaries so when your ALO asks for help, you can easily answer no. Ask your spouse or your significant other for input. Make sure you're together on these decisions. Find a boundary buddy who can help you stay firm but loving. A boundary buddy is someone who knows your values, respects you, and can talk you off the wall when you want to give into your ALO's demands in a weak moment.

Create a pre-planned list. It might look something like this:

I will say no to the following requests from my addicted loved one:

- Will you bail me out?
- Can I live with you for a while?
- Will you give me money for a hotel room?
- Can I use your car?
- Will you give me money for rent?

Having a "no" plan will conserve your energy and help you stay focused. If you know what you'll do, you won't spend time belaboring whether you'll help or not. You will still feel emotional tugs because you care, but if you discuss these decisions with your spouse and you've thought them through, pre-planning will help you enforce them.

Decision Automation: What decisions will you pre-decide?

_____

_____

_____

_____

Attention Allocation: How will you reallocate this attention toward your Boon?

_____

_____

_____

_____

Notes from the All-Mighty Mom Tribe

Brooke

To focus on conserving energy, I make my bed and exercise every day. I also pet my dogs several times every day. They bring a great deal of stress relief. I have a list of things I need to accomplish with three calendars to keep up with everything. A family in my community needs extra attention, so I take their little girls for art dates once a month. I sit on the board of a nonprofit that is working to bring a homeless shelter and transitional housing to our town. I can't emphasize enough the importance of a girl tribe. Mine is very diverse, from hippie party girls to those who wear the choir robe on Sunday. Truthfully, I dearly love all of them and feel blessed to have these souls in my life.

DAY 16

Assess Your Pain

Without pain, there would be no suffering.
Without suffering we would never learn from our mistakes.
To make it right, pain and suffering is the key to all windows,
without it, there is no way of life.

—Angelina Jolie

Welcome to the second half of the book! By now you've realized that being the mom of an addicted loved one is emotionally painful, and we have a lot of work to do in our own recovery. Have you heard the saying, "Pain is inevitable; suffering is optional?" We don't want to linger in the pain, but if we stay stuck, unable or unwilling to do our work, we could suffer for a long time. Maybe you already have. That's chronic pain.

What's the difference between acute pain and chronic pain?

When we don't take time to heal, chronic pain becomes inevitable. Moms of addicted loved ones who stay stuck in the misery choose to experience this endless pain every day. These moms sacrifice peace for suffering and live a life of unproductive inaction that often leads to loss of sleep, finances, and relationships.

Acute pain, on the other hand, brings significant breakthroughs. When moms embrace the pain, recognize it, and choose to find a way to recover, their suffering is short term. They're committed to becoming unhackable.

It's natural to try to avoid the pain, but choosing a life of focus means turning toward pain rather than away from it and locking onto *your* fight, not everyone else's. Unhackability means understanding and defining your pain, leaning into it, learning from it, and letting it go. By directing your focus toward your pain, you can work to resolve your problems and begin to close the gap between you and your Boon. If you don't realize you have pain, or if you're miserable and don't know why, it's time to figure it out.

Last month in the Tribe, one mom wanted to try something different. Exhausted from living in chronic emotional pain and trying to help her addicted daughter, nothing ever changed. The care team sisters listened to her with understanding and empathy and coached her toward making a few difficult decisions, including letting her daughter stay in jail instead of bailing her out.

Her daughter continued to call from jail and say things like, "Get me out of here. You don't love me. You never cared." Our mom was a wreck. She doubted her decision. With the group's support, we talked her through the crisis. She gave her daughter encouragement while she served her sentence. Eventually her daughter was released and found a job. She worked two weeks before she started having problems again and ended up homeless and jobless.

During this difficult time, this mom worked at maintaining her boundaries. When her daughter could talk coherently and agreed to work on her recovery, her mom listened, empathized, and affirmed her positive choices. When her daughter started talking nonsense and acted like she was using, her mom told her to call back when she was sober. Mom always expressed her love for her daughter before hanging up.

After a few months, they found her daughter on the streets in need of help. Police took her to a mental health facility, and after several weeks, she was diagnosed with schizophrenia.

Today our mom and daughter understand more about the underlying cause of her daughter's addiction and are seeking psychiatric help. Their relationship has blossomed. The daughter is taking her medication and learning about her mental health disorder. Her mother understands she had to go through this acute pain to stop the bleeding, the chronic pain. She went through so much turmoil before her daughter found help, but now she's at peace. Her temporary acute pain was worth it to get to the other side of her chronic pain.

We can't make choices for our loved ones, but we can learn how to respond to them differently. Doing the same thing repeatedly and expecting the same results doesn't work.

Peace of mind comes when we take time to understand ourselves and assess our pain. After we see our need for change, we can try to understand or motivate others to change.

Symptoms of Emotional Pain

It's important to understand our pain: where it comes from, what contributes to keeping it in place, how it affects you and those you love, and what to do about it going forward. If you refuse to acknowledge your pain, burying it instead, it will fester like a boil. You'll always feel it, and it will steal your joy, but it will never come to a head.

What can you do to identify your pain points and lean into them? Working with a therapist has helped me. When our pain stems from years of dealing with trauma, it's best to work with a therapist. If you've done that work and want to move into improving your future, I highly recommend working with a coach who can speak truth into your recovery plan.

Symptoms of emotional pain can include the following feelings:

- deep sorrow, sadness, or depression
- grief
- intense distress
- loneliness and isolation
- negative emotions
- panic
- rage
- shame

I used to think my son's addiction was partly my fault. I felt sorry for him, but pity always led to enabling. I helped him with things he could have done for himself. It made me feel good; however, I didn't build his self-esteem; I sent the message, "You can't do this, but I can."

Do you assume blame for your child's addiction? Does that pain get in the way of a healthy relationship with your child? If so, let me encourage you. There is no such thing as a perfect parent. If addiction were a parenting flaw, then every child would have an addiction because every parent is flawed.

When we take on our adult children's problems, we don't have time to work through our own problems. We remain locked in havoc, unable to see hope or achieve our recovery. When we allow others to solve their own problems and resolve difficult issues, we give them the power and motivation to change. This frees us to live our life and achieve our Boon.

CLOSE YOUR GAP DAY 16: ASSESS YOUR PAIN

For today's mission, journal these steps and questions.

Three Steps to Overcoming Pain

1. Determine the source of your pain. What obsessive thoughts keep you up at night, take you off task, or get in the way of your fun? Identify that pain.
2. Discover a way to lean into this problem so you can grow. How can you reframe this pain for growth potential? What will it take for you to overcome this pain? Do you need to forgive yourself or someone else?
3. Set a goal for how you will cope with this pain to grow and share it with an accountability or success partner.

Engage with the following questions:

- Up until now, how have you undermined your pain? Or if you leaned into it, what repeatable steps did you use to give yourself permission to heal?
- Up until now, how have you let your emotional pain get in the way of your healing and growing? Describe how letting go of this pain will help you achieve your Boon.

Notes from the All-Mighty Mom Tribe:

Brooke

Journaling has been a great tool for understanding myself and exploring the emotional pain I frequently feel. Pouring my thoughts onto paper relieves the anguish inside my soul. It's almost as if "seeing" the thoughts helps them occupy less brain space.

One a month, I write with a therapist who is my friend. Each of us throws out a writing prompt, and then we write for ten minutes. The only rule is that our pencil must be moving the entire ten minutes.

After writing, we read our piece out loud. The listener cannot judge or comment. Our only response can be "I can relate," or "I didn't quite get that."

This exercise has proven to be very cathartic and emotionally soothing. It helps me recognize the things that occupy my thoughts. I aspire to acknowledge and address the pain so I can move forward with less emotional weight. I cannot control my addicted loved one, but I can choose to focus on regulating myself.

***

Lucretia

To embrace my pain, my hurting heart, and my runaway thoughts, I must be consistent in my study time with the Lord. My Bible, devotionals, prayer book, and journal keep me grounded and encouraged as I live out my purpose of giving others hope. I also meet with accountability friends over coffee or lunch a couple of times a month. Nature walks, especially near water, calm me. I've had to be intentional about my daily choices so I can experience joy. Being in recovery is a choice—my choice—and I feel so much better.

DAY 17

Open Your Eyes

*When you begin to become conscious, more aware, when
your eyes begin to open, the first thing you see is how
deluded you are and how much
you're holding onto that which makes you suffer. This is, in
many ways, the most important step: Are you willing to be
aware?*

—Adyashanti

In Day 16, we leaned into our pain. Today, we're going to embrace our faith. Why? Because faith is the opposite of fear. Where there is faith, we find hope.

Look around your room right now and count how many red objects you see. Do this for two minutes. How many did you count?

Without looking around the room again, how many *green* objects did you see?

You probably didn't see many green things because you weren't looking for them. You were looking for red things.

We see what we're looking for.

The same is true with sound. If we're not listening for something, we might miss it. Constantly, negativity and anxiety keep us from seeing the positive events, people, and circumstances in our lives.

Fortunately, we can change our focus. We can start looking for the green things in our lives now—those things we are grateful for.

A good example is when our addicted loved one says something like, "I quit using for five days but relapsed." We can respond with, "You took a stab at something difficult. Well done," rather than, "Five days wasn't very long. Bummer."

Do you see this little shift? We're affirming the positive instead of seeing only the failure.

Napoleon Hill, author of *Think and Grow Rich*, said, "Our minds become magnetized with the dominate thoughts we hold in our minds . . . these 'magnets' attract to us the forces, the people, and the circumstances of life which harmonize with the nature of our dominating thoughts."[22]

Looking at the chaos keeps us from seeing hope. In my example, the addicted child's attempt to change was a positive step. If we accentuate the negative, not only will we continue to see the negative, but our child will too.

If we want to be different, we need to see differently. We must change our dominating thoughts so we stop attracting things we don't want in our lives. When we open our mind's eye and focus on the positive, we'll see everything we need.

> Your eyes can only see and our ears can only hear what our brain is looking for.
> —**Dan Sullivan**

What Is Sensory Overload?

I always loved children, but as I approached my forties, I discovered I needed a complete hysterectomy. My child-bearing days were over.

One August evening, while walking with my husband, I experienced a calling I immediately shared with him. "There's a girl out there who needs us. I don't know where, but I feel called to adopt. She's already been born. We have to go find her."

My husband laughed. He thought my calling would go away, but it didn't.

Two years later, we traveled to Russia to adopt our daughter, Olivia. Her birthday is August 25, 1995, close to the day I had the calling.

After living in an orphanage for twenty-five months, Olivia was developmentally delayed. We expected that, but we didn't expect her sensory defensiveness.

The first experience happened before we left Russia. While staying in a hotel room waiting for our paperwork, Olivia became tired and threw herself back on the hotel's concrete floor. Her head made a cracking sound. The look on her face told us she had never experienced this before. We guessed she'd always sat on a padded surface, maybe a playpen or a mattress. She only threw herself down like that twice. She learned quickly.

When we returned to the states, Olivia flew into sensory overload many times. On each occasion, she would flap her hands in excitement and almost hold her breath. She did it when her bare feet touched the grass, when she bounced on the trampoline, when we brushed her body (an intentional therapy to stimulate touch), when she rode in the grocery cart, and when we pushed her on a swing.

If the experience was too intense, Olivia would cry, and we had to stop. The sound of running bath water caused intense anxiety from sensory overload, so we gradually added the water to the tub, then dipped her toes one at a time. Eventually, she overcame her fear of water and performed somersaults off the diving board by the time she turned three.

Olivia also overcame her sensory defensiveness, but it took time, intentionality, and an occupational therapist. By gradually adding sensory details to her life, we slowly helped her focus on coping with stimuli.

Many moms are trying to cope with sensory overload in their lives. I experienced an overload last week. As I attempted to follow an enchilada recipe, two puppies rolled around the kitchen, biting and barking, and my granddaughters argued. Meanwhile, the now twenty-five-year-old Olivia stopped by to talk to me about a problem with her coworker. A barrage of sounds and smells surrounded me. Everyone wanted something, mostly my attention. I couldn't focus on anything. It was pure chaos.

Moms of addicted loved ones often have many tasks to complete at one time; they can feel like our young Olivia. Imagine if we giggled and waved our hands up and down during these chaotic moments. Maybe our families would understand they needed to back off.

How do we tap into our superhuman ability to focus during these times when we can't hear ourselves think?

According to Dr. Lee Angle:

Our bodies are filled with sensors that detect temperature, touch, sound, and vibrations. This information is gathered and transmitted by our nervous system to the brainstem. Once there, a filter sorts the information and decides what's important and what's not. Then it sends the information to the cortex of the brain when it makes a decision and responds accordingly.[23]

This filter is called the reticular activating system (RAS). The RAS is a bundle of nerves at the base of the brainstem that filters sensory information. When the RAS functions properly, it provides an environment for a child, or mom, to focus, learn, and follow instructions. When the RAS malfunctions, a typical environment can become overwhelming. In Olivia's circumstance, she couldn't handle overstimulation and was unable to focus. She had a sensory processing disorder.

Understanding how to use your RAS filter is necessary for becoming Unhackable. Your RAS filter prevents information overload.

The conscious brain processes about forty bits of information a second. That might sound impressive until we realize the subconscious brain processes over 11 million bits of information a second.[24]

That estimate is conservative. In his book, *Evolve Your Brain*, Dr. Jo Dispenza says, "The brain processes 400 billion bits of data every second."

What does all this brain information have to do with becoming an Unhackable Mom? Everything. Your RAS filter is super important, and how you can leverage it is even more important.

Your RAS filter is neutral. It can be your worst enemy or your best friend. If you tell it to look for all the negative road-blocks, barriers, and objections, then your brain will do an awesome job of gathering information that confirms your worst fears. It will tell you your child will never recover, and you'll never reach your Boon, so you'll stop trying before you start. You won't see hope.

What you process through your RAS filter becomes your reality. If you see your child, or yourself, as failures and losers, you'll repel successful people. After all, why would successful people want to associate with losers? We can't control who our children hang out with or what they think, but we can choose to see things differently, so we attract others who see the glass half full.

If you're like most people, your Boon might still be blurry. That's okay. Acknowledge your fear. You might be afraid you can't achieve it because you've never tried this before. Your Boon is new. It's change, and change isn't easy.

Think of it this way: You have a choice, a fork in the road. You can go right or left. One path strengthens your fears; the other boosts your faith and invites change. Remember, you don't have to change everything at once; you only need to continually take a baby step at a time.

FEAR + RAS FILTER = MORE FEAR
FAITH + RAS FILTER = MORE FAITH

You'll always reinforce what you focus on. Neuropsychologist Donald Hebb discovered that pathways in the brain are formed and reinforced through repetition. "Neurons that fire together wire together."[25]

To avoid seeing the reasons why your Boon will never come true, don't focus on the negatives. If you want doors to open for your idea and opportunities to come your way, focus on those. When you see them, express gratitude. When we practice our faith, we become a stronger version of ourselves.

CLOSE YOUR GAP DAY 17: OPEN YOUR EYES

- List the fears that make you think your Boon won't come true. What if none of those fears come true? Write the opposite of those fears. What if your Boon does come true? Journal what your life would look like.

- List five things you commit to looking at differently.

- List five things you will stop looking for.

- How will resetting your RAS filter move you closer to achieving your Boon?

Notes from the All-Mighty Mom Tribe

Brooke

Since my son has been revived from an overdose several times, I worry that he will use a substance that will kill him one day. It's a legitimate concern.

Many days I am so scared I have panic attacks, night terrors, and exhausting loop thinking. Fear of my son dying has caused me to be unable to live well.

Today I am choosing to focus on this moment. My son is alive right now. He has every opportunity to change if he wants. He also has my blessing to exercise free will and live the way he chooses.

I will love him no matter what. Love and fear are opposites, so I am lavishing love on my tortured adult child and believing the Lord will comfort all of us no matter what's next.

***

Lucretia

The fear that holds a space in my mind is that Joshua will have a very bad day or days, and his anxiety level will go through the roof. I fear he won't be able to control his anger and either go off on someone and get in trouble, slip, or relapse.

Another fear stems from so many people depending on me. I'm afraid I won't have time to do the things I want to do like take courses, workshops, and coaching classes. I'm helping my elderly parents move right now, and it's taking longer than my mind and body can take.

Five things I can look at differently:

1. Turning my fears into positive self-thoughts and talk.

2. Continuing to learn to listen to God and follow His step, give Him room to work in my life, and not try to control everything. Psalm 32:8 speaks to me: "I will instruct you and teach you the way which you should go; I will counsel you with My eye upon you." (NRSV)
3. Finding someone to help me with my elderly parents.
4. Saying, "no." I don't have to say yes to everything and everyone.
5. Putting my self-care higher on my priority list. I can't work out three hours a day, but I can walk two times a day and drink more water.

Five things I'm going to stop looking for:

1. Ways to fix my children's life issues.
2. Things to say. I will only listen when they call.
3. Answers. I will use questions to help them figure out their own problems.
4. Chaos. I will add rest and relaxation to my to-do list.
5. Unhealthy food. I will find more yummy keto recipes.

To reset my RAS Filter is to continually keep my Boon in front of me, to focus on the next step and not the whole staircase, to set my thoughts on positive ways of achieving my Boon and take action. My Boon is to grow my life coaching business by speaking and coaching 5,000 ladies by 2025, inspiring moms of addicted loved ones to become unstuck and take the next right step in their own recovery. My passion is to encourage and equip other women on their journey of self-care in whatever season they are going through.

DAY 18
Amplify Your Impact

Every choice you make has consequences;
certain losses, certain gains, possible losses, and possible gains.
Decide if the possible gains are worth the certain losses,
and if they are, find the courage to leap.
If they aren't, make peace with and appreciate the choice
not to risk what you already have.

—Doe Zantamata

A panic attack can make a person feel dizzy. It's like that moment right before surgery when they put the mask over your face. Your body begins to shut down, and you have no control. You gasp for air, but it doesn't bring more energy. Your body goes limp, and you think, *There's nothing I can do. I'm going to lose consciousness.*

I had one of these attacks days after my dog died. Out of nowhere, I felt like I was losing consciousness and then went limp. My doctor told me my excessive crying triggered a response like depression or a panic attack. I didn't understand, but I knew I never wanted to feel like that again. With time and medication, I overcame that attack. But I never forgot it.

The worry of my son's addiction brought back those feelings of panic. The heavy, dizzy feeling scared me. Since I recognized the signs, I worked to stop the attack in its tracks using coping strategies: breathing exercises, visiting my doctor, and exercising.

Worry can wreck our bodies. We envision our children lying in hotel rooms, overdosed. We picture them in jail, beaten, or homeless on the streets. When this happens, our body releases a stress hormone called cortisol. It's equivalent to our computer having so many windows open that it crashes. Our bodies can crash too, and when they do, our impact is compromised.

We can let go of this worry, but first, we need coping strategies.

Unhackable Impact Equation ©

When the thoughts swirling in our minds send us crashing, like our computers, we need to close some programs so we can have maximum impact on other projects. How will you shut off worrisome thoughts so you can focus on you, your goals, and your Boon?

One strategy is the Do It, Delegate It, or Dump It Strategy. Kary Oberbrunner calls it the Unhackable Impact Equation.©

DO IT	You do it!
DELEGATE IT	Somebody else does it.
DUMP IT	No one does it.
DELAY IT	You put off thinking about it until your "Worry Time."

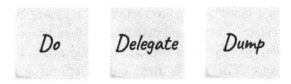

Do Delegate Dump

Do It

Examine your worry. Is there something you can do about the situation? List the possible solutions you could implement yourself. Which one makes the most sense? Try not to get hung up on the perfect solution. Choose one option and execute that task.

It's important to focus on those things you can control instead of what you can't change. One mom, worried about her heroin-addicted daughter, chose to plan her daughter's funeral. She felt like planning the funeral was the only thing she could control. It helped her. Thankfully, her daughter is many years in recovery now, but her mom focused on what she could do instead of what she couldn't do.

Delegate It

Will giving responsibility to someone else help your stress level?

At one time in our son's addiction, I didn't want to handle communication with him and our daughter-in-law because it hacked every energy byte in my body. They wanted to see their children, but because they weren't sober, I didn't want to put the girls in that situation. My emotions made it difficult to find the right words. My husband agreed to take over the communication. Delegating this helped me immensely. I no longer felt stuck in the middle.

Some moms give God control. They say, *I will let go and let God. He loves my children more than I do. He has a plan. Only he is in control.* This coping mechanism helps us stay focused on those things we can control. It's liberating to give our worries to God.

Even though some parts of our relationship with our child must be delegated so we can have the greatest impact, I strongly recommend studying motivational interviewing skills to keep communication with your loved one open. We must let go of the chaos, pain, shame, and blame but never our child. Look for a course or join a support group that teaches implementation of change talk when interacting with our addicted loved ones.

Dump It

Our loved ones will call us names, hang up on us, and get angry when we refuse to give them money, fix their cars, bail them out, and allow them to live with us. It's important to realize the negative energy doesn't come from our child. It comes from the addiction and the enemy. We must not take their words personally. We are doing the best we can, so we must find a way to dump the drama.

Tuning into your emotions might help shed light on why you're stuck or worried about uncertainty. Understanding your feelings can help you start to accept them, even when they're uncomfortable or don't make sense.

I don't want you to end, or dump, your relationship with your addicted loved one. But we can dump the feelings, the worry, and the guilt. It is difficult, if not impossible, to interact with a person when they're under the influence of a controlled substance. Fortunately, it is possible to love them enough to wait for a better opportunity to communicate. Which brings us to the last part of this strategy.

Delay It

Often, we'll have to wait for our addicted loved one to have a clear day to have a conversation. Guilt eats at us when we feel like we've given up on our child; however, when we label our silence a delay, we start to understand we haven't given up; we've saved the communication for a time when emotions won't ruin the relationship.

Another delay strategy a counselor recommended years ago is called Worry Time. Here's how it works:

1. Choose a day and time to designate as your Worry Time. For example, Tuesdays at noon.

2. During the week, when you feel stress rising, stop and jot down a few words about the worrisome thought. Tell yourself you'll worry about the problem later.

3. Let that worry go with the assurance you will revisit the thought next Tuesday at noon.

4. Since burying feelings and worries becomes unhealthy, on Tuesday at noon, review your weekly journal. Are you still struggling with the things you wrote? If so, allow yourself to worry. Journal your new thoughts. What will you do with this worry? Return to the Do It, Delegate It, Dump It philosophy.

5. If you're no longer worried about those thoughts, congratulate yourself on your resiliency and consider the things that have changed. You might notice a coping pattern you hadn't realized you possessed.

This exercise has the potential to change your perspective on worry. You'll build resilience and learn how to manage your other stressful thoughts.

CLOSE YOUR GAP DAY 18: AMPLIFY YOUR IMPACT

Follow these steps to amplify your impact:

- **Identify.** Grab some sticky notes. On each one, write a worry or unresolved issue that hacks you when making decisions or working toward your Boon. Give yourself time to list them. These could be big or small issues. Don't rush the process. Play calm instrumental music and give yourself time to write them all down.

- **Arrange.** Spread the sticky notes out on a table or wall. Look over your worries. How are they hacking you? Consider how much time each day you let these issues steal your energy.

- **Decide.** To amplify your impact, you'll need to close these windows. Create three columns for your sticky notes: Do—Delegate—Dump. Crumble each sticky note in the Dump column, and Do or Delegate the rest.

- **Delay.** During the week, allow Worry Time to help you sort new worries. Then once a month or more, sort each continued worry using the Do It, Delegate It, Dump It theory.

Notes from the All-Mighty Mom Tribe

Lucretia

If I let my thoughts run crazy, my anxiety goes through the roof, and my health is in jeopardy. I remember this quote: "If you don't take care of your own wellness, you will be taking care of your illness." Self-care matters!

My son, Joshua, got out of prison after two years and entered a transition house. He got there on a Friday afternoon and had the whole weekend to chill. With no staff to watch over him, he went a little wild. He didn't do anything bad; he just wandered outside for hours. He walked everywhere and bought a new phone, snacks, shoes, and sunglasses. He did those things he couldn't do while he waited for freedom.

When he returned to the transitional home, they confiscated his phone for a week. He hadn't read the rules of the house and had been gone too long.

I didn't know any of this, and after not hearing from him for a few days, my thoughts declined. My fear was that he messed up and would go back to prison.

Thankfully, that didn't happen. As punishment, he had to write an essay about why he was in prison, what his focus should be after his release, and what he was feeling.

He must be accountable to them, not me. I cannot police him.

When he finally called to tell me why I hadn't heard from him, I was relieved. He sounded humbled and had met with the director and the therapist.

We moms always think the worst. I was mad at myself because I allowed my thoughts to go places they shouldn't have gone. It's hard to stop, hard to cut off those negative thoughts, but I will do better. I will take my thoughts captive.

***

Pam Lanhart

Family Addiction Recovery Coach, Founder and Director of Thrive Family Recovery Resources, and Author of *Praying Our Loved One Home*

As I think about the shift that determined how I would walk through this journey with my loved one, I realize there were a few profound moments.

The first came as I sat in a pastor's office. He said to my husband and me, "Are you going to be right for the sake of justice, or will you love for the sake of relationship?"

Jesus paid the price for justice on the cross. I didn't have to be right. I didn't have to win. I was called to love. Because love never fails.

The second was when I grasped the true meaning of "do no harm." One thought drove me: *If my loved one got sober and ended up in recovery, would he want to have a relationship with me?*

I know too many families who have been ripped apart by addiction. When the ALO gets healthy, he decides he can't be around his toxic family. I didn't want to be that "toxic" family member. I wanted my son to know we would always be a safe space for him to come whenever he needed support.

I determined I wouldn't support the addiction, but I would support anything positive he chose to do, and regardless of his choices, I would always love him.

Finally, I knew death was part of the disease. If my son died, I wanted no regrets. What would that look like? Would he know he was loved? I asked myself, "If this were the last interaction with my loved one, could I live with what I'd said and done?"

That began my recovery. I knew I had to change. No expectations. No judgment. Radical love.

I have not been perfect. I have not always done things right. But I have done the best I could with the information and skills I had at the time.

I will keep moving forward. Our lives depend on it.

I am Pam Lanhart, and I am a person in long-term recovery from the effects of the disease of addiction.

***

October 23, 2021, Pam Lanhart lost her precious son, Jake. She wrote this:

Today our "what if" happened. Today our sweet son, our beautiful boy, was overcome by the disease of addiction.

We know that he touched many lives, and we ask for three things:

If you are struggling with an SUD, or if you are a friend of Jake's and you are in this battle, the greatest way you can honor Jake's life is to reach out for help.

If you are in the field, boots on the ground doing this work, keep doing it. Don't let this loss discourage you. Instead, double down to help those who are lost in this disease.

If you are a parent, spouse, or loved one of someone who suffers, call them tonight. Reach out to them and tell them you love them. Hug them even if they are using. Even if they seem unaware or don't care. Treat them with human dignity. Show them they are loved, not just in words but in kindness, compassion, and empathy.

Jake fought hard for his sobriety. I know many of you will grieve with us over this loss. We will honor our son by continuing the important work we do every day.

And please know this: We do not grieve as those who have no hope. Our hope has always been and will always continue to be in Christ alone.

"Go rest high on the mountain. Son, your work on earth is done. Go to heaven a-shoutin' love for the Father and the Son."[26]

DAY 19

Activate Your Diet

We don't see things as they are; we see them as we are.
—Anaïas Nin quoting the Talmud

This is the final day in the Focus module. By now you have learned how important it is to stay focused on yourself and what you want so you can recover from the addiction chaos in your life and achieve your Boon. Today, I'll share another tip to help you stay focused. This is the DIET approach. (I promise not to make you eat tofu and brussel sprouts every day unless you want to.)

You are the most important person you'll ever lead. How you view yourself is more important than how much money you have or who you know. It's more powerful than your intelligence because your self-esteem influences what you do and who you become. Therefore, it greatly influences your Boon.

Often, we are our own worst enemy. We let self-doubt get in the way of making achievements.

How do you see yourself? Are you a critic, complainer, caretaker, consumer, or creator?

Let's examine the Focus Framework, created partially by Kary Oberbrunner.

FOCUS FRAMEWORK©

IDENTITY	INPUT	OUTPUT
Consumer	No filter (Everything Goes In)	Nothing
Critic	No filter (Everything Goes In)	Nothing
Complainer	No filter (Everything Goes In)	Nothing
Caretaker	No filter (Nothing Goes In)	Nothing
Creator	Filter (Some Things Go In)	One Thing

Here's how this framework breaks down:

Identity

This is how you see yourself. Your identity influences your actions. Speakers speak. Writers write. Joggers jog. Teachers teach. In the example above, consumers consume, critics criticize, complainers complain, caretakers give their time to others, and creators create. How do you see yourself?

Who you are makes a difference in how you see things. When I took the Strengths Finder test, optimism ranked as my top strength, so I see the glass half full when others see it half empty because that's who I am.

> Life doesn't give us what we want. It gives us who we are.
> —**Anonymous**

You were created for a purpose, and when you find that, you understand where you need to place your focus. Knowing your purpose helps you focus on how to minimize distractions so you can recover and achieve your Boon.

Input

This is what you take in. Consumers, complainers, caretakers, and critics don't have any filters. They don't know how to say no to the distractions that hack their focus.

Consumers consume everything at random times and in random ways without focusing on achieving much of anything.

Critics input everything, causing skepticism. As we said on Day 14, your focus determines your input. Critics can only see what's wrong and spend their time and energy finding fault in things that don't matter.

Like the critics, a complainer's input produces negativity. They spend their energy complaining, never creating solutions or growing themselves so they can be a part of the Kingdom's solutions. Journalist Paul Brian researched the effects of complaining. He discovered the most cutting-edge research out of places like Stanford University shows that complaining opens the floodgates for stress hormones that bathe your neurons in bad chemicals. You start to find it harder to make decisions, solve problems, and understand situations realistically because everything becomes "amped up" by stressful, anxiety-producing feelings.[27]

Caretakers input everything and see only problems, so they spend their time helping others, putting out fires, spiraling in chaos and don't know how to say no to accomplish their dreams.

Creators, on the other hand, have a filter. As a result, they only allow things into their lives that help them achieve their Boon. When they plan their day, they filter out thoughts and activities that don't help them achieve their goals. Helping others and contributing might be part of what they accomplish, but they run those tasks through a purpose filter first to qualify them. Everything they do, even helping others, will fit their Boon creation.

Output

This is what you put out. Consumers and critics aren't putting anything out there. Consumers are too busy consuming — high calorie food, video games, TV series, and other media. Critics stay busy watching others, criticizing their performance. Complainers focus on everything wrong with others as well as themselves. They stay stuck in not producing anything. Caretakers have a heart for others. They help them get what they want, which sounds commendable, but because they struggle with saying no, it doesn't help them or the ones they care for live in their sweet spots. They have huge hearts but never pursue their own dreams.

Some moms might have a Boon to help others. Care*givers* use their helping skills as a part of their Boon. They help others get what they need so they can be transformed into the best person possible. In that case, they're creators too. Creators are focused on achieving something: their Boon.

CLOSE YOUR GAP DAY 19: ACTIVATE YOUR DIET

Before reading this book, how did you see yourself?
___Consumer ___Critic ___Complainer ___Caretaker
___Creator

With your new awareness, how do you now see yourself?
___Consumer ___Critic ___Complainer ___Caretaker
___Creator

If you aren't where you want to be yet, how will you refocus? What steps will you take?

The next step is creating your DIET. You have done so much already. You know your Boon and the benefit it will bring, so you're headed in the right direction. Your DIET will help you hyper-focus.

D = Determine where you want to go.

Write your Boon again. I'm praying you have more clarity today than you did on Day 2 when you first heard the word Boon and started thinking about what this could be for you. The more defined our Boon becomes, the clearer we will be able to see where we want to go.

I = Identify who's getting the results you want.

Do you know someone doing what you want to do? If so, spend time studying this person. How can you connect with him or her? If possible, interview him or ask him to mentor or coach you.

For instance, when I wanted to appear on more podcasts, I found a man who offered a course and coaching on how to connect. I joined his group and learned his success secrets. Remember, my Boon is to empower one million moms, so I'm always running everything through that filter. Will getting on ten high-profile podcasts help me spread my message? Yes!

Maybe your Boon is to achieve a more peaceful life. Look for a mom in our Tribe who has a peaceful mindset. Suppose you find someone coping well with her addicted loved one and finding ways to connect with her child. How awesome would it be if you reached out to her and asked her to help you develop a positive mindset or be your personal mentor? I have a feeling she would be honored.

Make a list of those positive people you want to study. Read each bio and read their business reviews. Private message others who know the person and ask questions. After you feel confident you want to know more about this person, reach out.

E = Eliminate the empty calories.

I love chips, pretzels, and Tostitos. I often crave them in the middle of the day. I also fancy a good game of sudoku and enjoy scrolling through Facebook, Instagram, and Pinterest.

What empty calories do you crave? How are those calories serving you? Typically, they bring extra pounds and slow me down. They don't give me energy. Unhackability doesn't happen by accident. We must want it. We must be intentional.

Make a list of your empty calories. When will you eliminate them? Now? Next week? Within the next twenty-four hours? How would your productivity increase if you limited your time on Facebook, Instagram, and Pinterest? Would you push through if you allowed yourself play time or empty calories only after you accomplished one step in your Boon? Today, for instance, I told myself I could watch TV only after I finished this chapter.

T = Turn your focus only after squeezing and applying every drop of value.

When we adopted Olivia, I wanted to be a stay-at-home parent, so I decided to write for magazines and books. Initially, I thought, *How hard could it be*? Now I laugh. It was wicked tough to write a best-selling novel and get published, but I did, many times.

The competitive side of me was determined to learn, so I looked for online writers' groups that shared tips and started following them. I went to conferences, workshops, and retreats. I studied fictional elements. I found one group that showed me how to gain followers, apply for contests, and learn the basics of writing fiction. I took college courses and made getting published my Boon. Every part of my day filtered through that goal.

When I wasn't doing something with Olivia, I was writing or communicating with best-selling authors. I became part of a crowd who helped me grow. I stayed with them until I felt I'd learned everything possible, then I moved on to find another treasure trove. This is what I want for you.

Commit to staying the course with the people you identified above. Stay with them until you've learned everything you need to learn, but don't forget to keep creating too.

I will turn my focus only after squeezing and applying every drop of value.

_____ Yes _____ No

Notes from the All-Mighty Mom Tribe
Brooke

I = Identify

The first step I took toward recovery was to join an Al-Anon group, and I forced myself to attend every week for a year. I found a wonderful group of ladies in that room, and they remain close to my heart now, many years later.

Dakota was one of my Al-Anon friends who became my hero. She was a treasured and unique soul who taught me how to live and die well.

I studied her because I noticed she had deep and meaningful relationships, was transparent, and real. I wanted what she had! She listened with a nonjudgmental ear and was kind to the depths of her soul. Dakota could express what she needed in a direct, unassuming way. That's a gift I have never experienced in another person. She was truly one of a kind.

Dakota enticed me to confide in her because she knew how to listen, silently but expressively. She had a depth of understanding and a strong faith in God and other people. I don't know that I have ever felt loved by anyone except her. She had the uncanny ability to make me feel seen, known, and understood in a way that no one before or after her has been able to replicate.

She fought many forms of cancer, and when she knew she was dying, she gathered all her friends together at her home. "Look over my personal belongings here. Take what you want to help you remember me," she said.

I took a fur coat, her wedding veil and gloves, a few sweaters, and a memoir of treasures she shared. She handed me an envelope before I left. Inside was a card, a large sum of money, and a note:

"Brooke,

"Thank you for the many laughs we've had in this insane asylum of the universe. (When things didn't make sense to her, she would say this phrase.)

"I am so glad we were able to walk this walk together to nurture and enjoy each other. I love you to the moon and beyond. You are my family. Use this money to take David on a trip."

A few days later, she told us it was time for her to go. She called hospice because the pain from her pancreatic cancer was overwhelming, and she wanted to be comfortable as she let go of this insane asylum of the universe.

Before the nurse sedated her, she gathered twenty-five of us, her friends, around the bed. We read her preferred Bible passages and told stories about our time with her. We laughed and cried, and everyone said goodbye. She passed several weeks later.

Months later, I took David, my grandson, to D.C. with the money she left me. I still have two of her cards in my windowsill.

I will love her forever, listen to her wisdom play in my head, and admire the person God chose to be my mentor and friend. Rest easy, Dakota. Thanks for teaching me about life, love, and the journey. My time with you will forever be a highlight in my story.

PART FOUR

Optimal Mom Performance

DAY 20

Find Your All-Mighty Mom Flow

The happiest people spend much time in a state of flow—
the state in which people are so involved in an activity
that nothing else seems to matter;
the experience itself is so enjoyable that people will do it
even at great cost,
for the sheer sake of doing it.

—Mihaly Csikszentmihalyi

Welcome to Part Four of this thirty-day process. In this section, you will learn how to optimize your performance by reaching your flow. Flow occurs when you are in the zone. You possess the ability to make decisions quickly and accomplish tasks and goals because your inner critic goes silent. You no longer have negative thoughts filling your brain. During flow you slow down long enough to positively impact your daily outcome.

Performing like an *All-Mighty Mom* simply means you're focused, you have a determination to heal, recover, and be the best you can be despite the distractions that accompany a child with an SUD.

Finding my *All-Mighty Mom* status includes intentionally and continually building a better relationship with the Almighty God, strengthening my faith, and learning how to lean on Him. Spending time in the Bible has helped me see opportunities and divine moments I wouldn't have otherwise noticed. Addiction is a spiritual battle, and to reach optimal performance, practicing my faith is a part of the solution for me. I pray it is for you too. Your Higher Power might be different than mine but equally important.

Flow might seem impossible. But flow can be experienced by anyone, anytime, anywhere, under the right conditions. I would guess you've already experienced flow in your life, and you can experience it again. You might not have realized it as flow, but once you learn more about it and how to achieve it, you will intentionally seek more. It's healthy and can help you achieve your Boon and leave your legacy.

To experience this flow state, we need to find ways that work for us. When I play the piano in privacy and create songs, all inhibition leaves. I can walk away from the experience in a peaceful state without a care in the world. When I write fiction, I become immersed in my character's lives, and I experience the same feeling. This is flow.

Mihaly Csikszentmihalyi was the first person to research flow. As a prisoner during World War II, he witnessed the pain and suffering of the people around him and became curious about happiness and contentment. In Csikszentmihalyi's words, flow is "a state in which people are so involved in an activity that nothing else seems to matter; the experience is so enjoyable that people will continue to do it even at great cost, for the sheer sake of doing it."[28]

Characteristics of Flow

When we're out of flow, we judge everything we're doing through a skewed filter. We tell ourselves we're not good enough, our idea will never work, or we'll never find peace. Outside of flow, our critic takes over. Flow is important because it allows us to act without over-thinking or self-editing everything we say and do.

Here's what happens when you are in flow:

You become totally absorbed. One mom in our Tribe shared that when she cleans houses, she turns on her favorite music and loses herself in the job. She's in her zone. Her mind focuses only on what she's doing and how she will get it done within a certain time period. She doesn't think about her addicted adult child. She doesn't worry about her grandchildren. She gets her work done with focus and flow.

You have extreme focus. As this mom focuses on cleaning every inch of the countertops and sweeping every corner, she doesn't see the problems in her world. Flow silences the negative chatter; she stays immersed in creating a clean-living space for her clients. A person in flow can achieve hyper-focused results almost effortlessly, without little thought to what they're doing.

You are unaware of time. Do you remember being young and in love? Spending time with your new boyfriend made an hour feel like a minute. Time passes similarly in flow. Part of flow for our house-cleaning mom is seeing each part of her job completed before she's done. She sees the future and loses track of time. Before she knows it, the job is done.

You concentrate on things you can control. Many things helped in my recovery. The first was realizing I was powerless over my child's choices, and only God is in control. The second was learning and embracing the three Cs. They allowed me to support my loved one and embrace my boundaries.

The Three Cs

- "I can't **cure** their addiction." Addiction is a chronic disease like diabetes or hypertension and requires guidance from a medical professional. I am not a doctor.
- "I didn't **cause** it." Our loved ones want to blame us, but that's because it's easier to blame us than to blame themselves.
- "I can't **control** it." Addiction is a biological disease that affects the brain's chemistry. There's nothing moms can do to control our children's actions. Letting go of the urge to try to control what our loved one does will help us find more productivity and flow. We'll be able to tackle those things we can change.

Your self-conscious rumination ceases. When Canada geese struck Captain Sully's plane causing double engine failure, he and all his passengers were heading for the Hudson River. In that moment, he went immediately into flow. He had spent his career developing the skills he needed to land the plane in the water. In his state of hyper-focused attention, all other thoughts ceased. His successful emergency landing was a result of these flow characteristics.

Your feel rewarded. Bringing value to others makes my heart swell. When I'm working for the good of others, I get into flow and don't think about my problems. Flow brings reward. When our mom finished cleaning her house for the day, she felt like she had accomplished something. Although her paycheck provided a reward, she had intrinsic reward too. Sometimes that feeling is priceless. When Captain Sully saved the people on the plane, I'm certain his heart swelled too. My goal to empower one million moms drives me to stay into flow. Each time I complete a chapter in this book, I experience an intrinsic reward.

Respond versus React

Distractions rob us from experiencing flow, so it's important to assess our distractions. Yours might be different from mine. But typically, moms of addicted loved ones fear their children will die of an overdose. That fear dominates thoughts and steals our flow patterns.

Learning how to *respond* to your ALO's actions instead of *reacting* will help you stay in flow without hacking your progress. This skill takes practice, but once you learn it, you'll be able to communicate with your loved one more effectively, feel calmer, and stay focused on accomplishing your Boon. This minor shift will help you sleep better, reduce your stress, and improve your relationship with your loved one.

When our ALOs get angry or find a way to blame us for their struggles, we tend to react without thinking; emotion and anger take over. Afterward, we feel guilty, which causes us to give in to our loved one. They get what they want, which removes all motivation to change, perpetuating the cycle.

Learning response techniques can interrupt the pattern:

Step 1: When you feel triggered by something your ALO did or said, pause.

Step 2: Take an intentional deep breath. Walk away if you must, or say, "I'll get back to you later about this."

Step 3: Assess your emotion in that moment. What set you off?

Step 4: What do you want? Keep your eyes on your overall goal instead of the immediate emotion.

Step 5: Respond when you're ready.

> Between stimulus and response there is a space. In that space is our power to choose our response. In our response lies our growth and our freedom.
> —**Viktor E. Frankl**

Responding rather than reacting keeps us in control and our emotions calm. It frees us from chaos. When we react, it's instinctive and in opposition to a situation or person. While responding is still a reaction, it's more thought out. Responding allows time to evaluate our goals. A response is engineered to produce a positive outcome.

Reactions have the potential to make the situation worse and leave us with regrets. They jumpstart the repeating thoughts cycle and keep us out of flow.

Look at the differences between reacting and responding:

Reactions are	**Responses**
Impulsive	Respect your core values
Instant	Are thought out
Said without thinking	Look at the long-term goal
Triggered by the past	Happen slower and after a pause
Regretted	Are honest and helpful
Defensive	Are expressed calmly

Expressing anger, frustration, and disgust with our loved ones only keeps them locked in shame and holds us in a stressful state that blocks flow. I want you to find flow because that's the place where you can accomplish the steps to your dream without anger, guilt, analyzing, hesitating, or worrying.

You'll be able to let go of unproductive thoughts and actions and love yourself as well as your ALO. You won't spend time trying to fix him/her, absorbing their pain, because your plan won't allow those types of interruptions.

CLOSE YOUR GAP DAY 20: FIND YOUR ALL-MIGHTY MOM FLOW

Life is full of lessons, but unless we take a moment to reflect on what we have learned, the moment will be wasted. By focusing on the lessons of your recovery, we're able to look back and see the process. Though we struggled, we found freedom. When we have a goal to stay in flow, we can learn and rise above the adversity. We can recover.

Understanding the necessary flow cycle of Struggle, Release, Flow, Recovery will help us get through our painful moments. On Day 22, we'll unpack the details of the four stages of the flow cycle.

For now, it's time to shift our perspective. Rather than viewing our struggle as a negative thing, let's begin to believe the struggle will help us reach your Boon.

List five reasons you're thankful for your struggles. For instance, the pain you've gone through already is helping you take the steps to be where you are today. What steps have you been thankful for? Below is my example:

> Without pain, there is no payoff. Without struggle, there is no Boon.
> —**Kary Oberbrunner**

1. If I hadn't gone through this addiction journey with my son, I wouldn't be helping other moms now, and I wouldn't be equipped to lead them.

2. I wouldn't have the close relationships I have with my granddaughters.

3. I wouldn't have met the women in this Tribe or other prominent people in the addiction world who made me a better person, a woman who is closer to God and my purpose.

4. Seeing addiction through my son's eyes has given me more compassion and understanding of people everywhere. I'm able to understand how important it is to be heard and understood. This journey has forced me to learn how to listen better.

5. Watching my child suffer has made me more compassionate and taught me about resiliency.

Now it's your turn. Write out five reasons why you're thankful for your struggles:

1.

2.

3.

4.

5.

Notes from the All-Mighty Mom Tribe
Sandy

If I hadn't gone through this journey, I might have believed I was in control of my life instead of God.

I would still believe people who are addicted to alcohol can stop anytime if they choose. I would not understand this is a brain disease and someone with alcohol use disorder is sick and needs medical treatment and therapy.

I would not feel the level of compassion and be able to give grace to the people who have suffered trauma and find themselves sick and stuck in the horrible cycle of addiction.

I wouldn't have become friends with or been supported by these amazingly strong women whom I admire for the way they are changing the world.

I wouldn't have learned to lean on God, seek him, write His promises on my heart, and have unwavering faith that He will never leave me!

***

Brooke

If I hadn't gone through this terrible struggle of addiction, I would not have an adopted family who has loved us through thick and thin.

I would not have a wild, whacky, and wonderful girl tribe because that would not have been necessary for me.

I would not have returned to church and established a deep belief in God.

I would not have my grandson who brings deep joy to my life.

I would not have a wonderful relationship with my step-children because my two boys would have been all I needed.

I would not be married to Howard.

I would be more judgmental toward people with addiction.

I would have no grasp of homelessness and would not have the deep sadness I feel toward those without homes.

I would not be on the board of a nonprofit that is attempting to address the concerns of homelessness in our town.

I would not be involved in the lives of my neighbor's children, Mattie and Grace.

I would not be teaching piano to my bonus granddaughters.

I would not study the Bible with women who feel my soul and sit still in the dark places.

I would not have been to Grief Recovery, where I made some deep discoveries about myself.

I would not be so involved in water sports because I wouldn't have needed to escape and sit in a peaceful place.

***

Lucretia

If I hadn't gone through this addiction journey with my son:

- I wouldn't have grown deeper with the Lord.
- I wouldn't have the relationship with Dylan, my granddaughter, and Ayden, my grandson.
- I wouldn't have learned and understood the stigma about addictions and the brain.
- I wouldn't have the compassion for the unseen moms of this crazy world of addiction.
- I wouldn't have sold my home and everything in it to move closer to my daughters.
- My daughter and son-in-law wouldn't have adopted Ayden.
- I wouldn't have let my business go and started another one.

- I wouldn't have found these moms to have hope with.
- I wouldn't have learned about how self-care is so important.

Without the struggle and pain, I wouldn't have set major boundaries.

DAY 21
Acknowledge Your Grief

My son's addiction has left a gaping hole in my life.
Falling in the hole or filling it up are my only options.
So, I'm taking steps to fill it.

—Sandy Swenson

As Moms, we struggle with the loss of dreams we have for our addicted loved ones. We never imagined them to be viewed as throw-aways by society. Some of us may have judged other adults for their poor life choices and thought of them as junkies (a word that makes me cringe) before we had a child with this disorder. Our perspectives have changed. Now we see the value in every person regardless of their addiction. We raised our child envisioning successful citizens with good jobs and families. This loss brings grief, and it's important to acknowledge it so we can heal.

Grief is a universal problem, yet not everyone talks about it. When we finally break out of our depression to talk to other moms who are struggling with this same loss, we don't feel alone. As we share similar yet unique stories, we find each person deals with grief differently. Some take longer to work through than others, but talking and recognizing our place in the process helps.

Below, I've listed the seven stages of grief. They can help us see where we are in the grieving process and affirm what we're feeling is normal.

The Seven Stages of Grief[29]

1. **Shock and denial:** In this part of the grief cycle, we think, *My child was brought up in a stable home and learned the "Just Say No" approach. There's no way he/she would mess with drugs or alcohol.*

2. **Pain and guilt:** We can't breathe or sleep because the loss is unbearable, and we think, *What did I do? How did I mess up my child's life so badly?* We might also think, *Why didn't I see this problem sooner?*

3. **Anger and bargaining:** In the next stage, we might take their using personally with thoughts like these: *How could my child do this to me? Maybe if I'm there for him and let him live with me, I can control and police his sobriety.*

4. **Depression:** *I'm so ashamed. Everyone knows about my child, so I'll stay home. Nobody understands.*

5. **The upward turn:** The stages of grief have died down, and we begin to experience calm. We're learning to accept that we can't control our loved one; we can only control ourselves.

6. **Reconstruction and working through:** We think, *Maybe I need to understand addiction better so I understand my child. After all, I want a better relationship with him.*

7. **Acceptance and hope:** *I can't control my child, but I can control my life. I am God's daughter. I have gifts and skills I can use to help fight addiction and the stigma in our world.*

Just like there are stages of grief, there are also stages of recovery for us and our children. When I studied the stages of addiction, I noticed the parallels between both.

Stages of Recovery for Moms

I created these stages of recovery based on what I've learned on my journey. Just like our addicted loved ones, moms can become addicted to micromanaging their children's problems and absorbing all their pain. Often moms don't see the similarities between their behavior and their child's addiction, but each person transitions through their recovery similarly.

First Stage: Grief, displaced guilt, anger, shame, obsessive thoughts that our child will die, difficulty understanding what's happening to our child. Possible enabling. Fixing. Covering for our child's actions.

Second Stage: Continued grief, awareness that something must change, learning how to let our child face the consequences of his or her actions, accepting the situation, learning about addiction and what our child must do on his or her own, realizing moms can't fix their addict's problems.

Third Stage: More grief, love for ourselves, searching for ways to find joy, reconnecting with our inner child, finding ways to self-care, making our wellness a priority. Loving our child despite his disease. Listening to him. Encouraging him into recovery without shame.

Fourth Stage: Still grieving but finding meaning in our recovery and grief. We're learning how to listen to our loved ones without trying to fix them by meeting them where they are and learning motivational interviewing skills to help motivate change in them and in us. We're finding a way to help moms in the earlier stages of grieving by making our mess a message.

How To Make Your Mess a Message?

Your journey is personal, so I can't tell you what to do or how you're going to make the biggest dent in helping others. I do know if we want to leave a legacy, we must be intentional. Use this exercise to increase your intentionality:

Reflect. Think about your life before your child had an SUD. What were you eager to try? Do you have a dream or interest you never pursued? Maybe you put your life on hold when your child became ill or cancelled your further education. Google "verses to help me reflect on my life" and ask God to help you remember what you wanted to do and show you what He wants you to do now.

Reimagine. What do you want out of recovery as you work through your grief? When pondering this question, think intellectually, spiritually, physically, creatively, socially, and emotionally. In each of these categories, where do you see yourself? How will you improve? Consider taking a college or online course, joining a book club or a Bible study group, learning pickleball or another sport, gardening, learning to play an instrument, taking a Zumba class, volunteering in your jail or homeless shelter, or taking an art class.

Replace. Your pain, grief, or worry doesn't help your loved ones. Those elements will not move your loved one into sobriety faster. It's imperative we take time to grieve, but as you work through the seven steps, think about what you'd like to substitute for the grief. What kind of growth would best replace the pain? How will you transform your mess into a message? Boundaries, self-care, and a growth plan make a great place to start. If you want to optimize your performance in life, balancing these three things will help you stay focused on you.

CLOSE YOUR GAP DAY 21: ACKNOWLEDGE YOUR GRIEF

It's time to write your recovery Boon Poem. You might think you can't write, but you'll be surprised. Your prose doesn't have to rhyme or be perfect. This is an exercise to help you heal. Write without stopping or editing. I find it helpful to use strong action verbs to describe my scenes.

Write your poem as you see yourself transitioning through the stages of grief and recovery above. Write about your life at the moment you realized your child was addicted. Describe your shock and detail the times you helped and how you cried each time the cycle continued. Share how you healed through the description of each stage. Use the three Rs to visualize where you were and where you want to be now. Think about where you want to be in your recovery a year from now. Don't hold back. Think big. Close out the enemy who wants you to believe you aren't enough, that you can't do the impossible. Don't edit any image that comes to mind.

Notes from the All-Mighty Mom Tribe

Michelle

Here is an example of a Boon Poem I wrote to illustrate how I see my screenplay. Writing this screenplay will give me another opportunity to empower one million moms of addicted loved ones. The movie is a part of my Boon that is yet to come, but I can see it happening. Having the vision motivates me to write the movie.

On the screen
The movie theatre seats filled with mighty women
Sisters in the trenches, mothers in agreement
About the pain and suffering
That comes from the trauma of a child in addiction.
Holding hands with heads high, they watch
The efforts of their suffering
Told through their stories
The stories of loss, love, and the enemy.
They watch the stories on the screen and
Cry for those afflicted
As if each story told is her own
One of holding on to the child she once knew
Without losing herself in the process.

***

Grieving The Loss of Someone Who Still Lives

by Lorelie Rozzano

When your loved one struggles with addiction, an internal battle plays out. On one hand, you're grateful that they're alive. On the other hand, you're mad as hell at them.

It's tragic watching drugs and alcohol turn someone you love into someone who breaks your heart. Losing someone to substance use disorder differs from losing a loved one to death. After all, your person is alive—kind of. But your loved one is not who they once were, and neither are you.

When your addicted loved one disappears from your life, or when they're too impaired to be effective, and they're committing suicide one fix at a time, your world turns upside down and inside out. You think about how it used to be and wonder where you went wrong. Sadness may occur every time you think about them, which is all the time.

Grieving the loss of someone who still lives is like riding a roller coaster. One moment you have hope, and the next, you're waiting for the dreaded phone call. It hurts when you realize you're not as important as you once were. You may find yourself wanting to avoid your emotional pain. Don't. Feel your sadness and grief. Don't judge it. If a voice in your head whispers—if they really loved me, they'd stop using—squash it. That voice is trying to take you away from your feelings. Sadness is a healthy emotion. Allow yourself to grieve. When you don't feel your feelings, they turn toxic and become misery fuelers like resentment, rage, and self-pity.

When you attach your well-being to your addicted loved one and make it your job to fix and rescue them, you become so caught up in their downward spiral you might fail to see the changes in yourself.

You've probably said, "if you love me, you'll stop using." But addiction has nothing to do with love. They're two different things. Chronic drug/alcohol use changes the chemical biology of the brain, and reward centers become strongly connected to their drug of choice (or addictive behaviors), and getting high becomes automatic. The addicted person's brain is hijacked, skipping the cerebral cortex, the area of the brain responsible for reasoning and impulse control, and instead reroutes through the old reptilian brain, the part of the brain responsible for survival. This part of the brain says,

"Get dope or die," and it's wired to choose the addiction above everyone/thing else.

Reasoning with your addicted loved one won't work either. Denial is a crucial symptom of this illness. Denial makes problems smaller than they really are. Denial minimizes the consequences while glorifying the good times. Addiction plays out through symptoms of delusion, denial, grandiosity, dishonest thinking, poor impulse control, and impaired judgment. If only love were enough. Unfortunately, it's not. The person you love has radically changed.

Addiction is like a brain injury similar to Alzheimer's and cancer in that it's progressive and can lead to death if untreated. While you can't love your addicted family member into wellness, there are things you can do to increase a successful outcome.

First and foremost, practice self-care. You can't help anyone if you're feeling angry and exhausted all the time. Instead of reacting to your pain, sit with it, feel it, deal with it, and heal it. Feelings that aren't shared and debriefed become unhealthy responses, like enabling.

Please know you're not alone. Many families are also in the same boat. Reach out for support. Connecting with safe, supportive people will increase your ability to cope, and you'll feel less impacted by your loved ones' actions. It might seem grim. But know that circumstances evolve, and now isn't forever.

When you empower yourself through education, boundaries, and support, the way you engage with your addicted loved one will change. Transformation doesn't happen in solitude and isolation but through connection with people sharing similar experiences.

Instead of waiting for the impaired thinker to see the light, lead the way because statistics show addicted persons have the best chance of succeeding when their families are educated and in recovery.

Lorelie Rozzano is an internationally recognized author and advocate. She's in long-term recovery and works in the field of mental health and addiction, helping patients and their families regain their health. Lorelie hopes the honesty found in her books, *Jagged Little Edges*, *Jagged Little Lies*, *Jagged No More*, and her children's book, *Gracie's Secret*, will inspire people to reach out for support. To learn more, visit jaggedlittleedges.com.

DAY 22

Unpack Your Cycle

*Chaos in the world brings uneasiness,
but it also allows the opportunity for creativity and growth.*
—**Tom Barrett**

Our goal is to heal, love ourselves and our children, and recapture our identity and purpose. Before we can master our positive flow habits, it helps to understand where we're getting stuck in chaos cycles. Only then can we live free and experience real flow.

When a child (adult or teen) has an SUD, many things happen to the family. As we reflect on each incidence, we see cycles of chaos with certain repeated patterns. See if the following patterns have been a part of the chaos in your family.

Five Stages of Chaos Cycles

1. **The problem or the event:** In the beginning of our child's SUD, he drinks with his friends in high school. We might think, *This is a phase. He'll outgrow it.* But

the next time, the event becomes more problematic. Something negative happens because of the substance use. He might lose his license, get arrested, be expelled, or lose his job.

2. **Chaos:** This problem or event triggers an immediate reaction in the family. Members become emotional and might exhibit shame, grief, anger, anxiety, fear, or other emotions.

3. **Role playing:** After each event, family members perform a role they're not aware of. Sometimes moms lecture. Dads and siblings typically play a different role. (You'll find a list of possible roles you play on Day 25.) Our addicted loved ones learn who plays which role and how to manipulate them, and the cycle continues. It's like a mobile turning over an infant's crib. The chaos cycle will keep going the same direction until one person decides to change his or her role. Only then will the cycle shift in a different direction. When someone finally interrupts the cycle, everyone must guard against shifting into the vacant role. When I decided to give up my lecture role, for example, my husband suddenly wanted to step in and play my part. Role transfer keeps the mobile moving and easily happens if we're not aware of the cycle.

4. **Temporary Return to Status Quo.** Typically, our role playing helps the addicted loved one escape the consequences of his using. If mom bails him out, dad fixes his car, or brother finds him a new job, things will seem okay, but not for long. Abstinence rarely lasts without a recovery plan. A person can't simply quit for the sake of quitting. Most addicted loved ones will fall into using again when they can't cope with a problem, or they face their trigger. Eventually a new

event will start the cycle again, and often there's a greater consequence.

5. **Victim mindset begins again**. Each time the addicted loved one gets in trouble, he gets more comfortable in the cycle. He has noticed if he listens to his mom lecture for a while and puts up with her ranting, then lets the rest of family rally and play their roles, they'll help him get out of the jam he got himself into. The addicted loved one learns to play the victim card. He tries to convince everyone the world is out to get him, or bad luck follows him. He wants us to believe he just needs a break, and he knows his mother will fall for this mindset. She might already feel this way about herself or her loved one. When a mom feels sorry for her child, she makes excuses for him and continues to try to fix the problem.

Instead, she needs to adopt the victor mindset we discussed on Day 3 and implement the proper listening skills to motivate change in her child without feeding the child's victim mindset or trying to take the consequences for her child. (Appendix B covers how to listen to others, and Appendix C covers motivating change.)

We can't heal from the chaos cycle until we understand our role and our family dynamics. Looking at our genogram can help.

Genograms

Genograms are pictures of a person's family relationships and history and provide a way to study family patterns. They can be helpful when working with a therapist to stop generational trauma, too. They help set the foundation for nurturing generational strengths and overcoming weaknesses. A genogram is like a family tree but includes the nitty-gritty details of how family members interact. Genograms include information about relationships and interactions between family members. A family tree might show us, for example, that Emily and Dave are siblings. A genogram would tell us they are related but emotionally distant from one another.

Sometimes genograms include information about several generations. They're an effective tool for therapists because patterns can be recognized that might otherwise be difficult to decipher.

Maybe you've already noticed a trend of marital trouble in your family's history. A genogram can highlight the pattern of anxiety and anger at the root of those marital problems. I encourage you to talk to a therapist about your genogram if you want to do the work to stop your family's cycle. There are other resources available if you're ready to do the work.

To see more on how to create a genogram, watch this YouTube video created by the Multicultural Family Institute: bit.ly/genogramvideo.[30]

Four Stages of the Flow Cycle

Now that you're aware of the possible chaos cycle in your family and how to study them, let's shift to the four stages of a flow cycle. Knowing this cycle will help you stay committed to achieving your Boon, despite the chaos that addiction brings to your life.

1. **Struggle:** In the first stage, you're gathering information, doing research, or brainstorming with friends about how you're going to tackle your task. Sometimes it can feel like you're trudging through mud because the progress feels slow.

If I use the example of writing a screenplay, I could say that I'm in the struggle stage. I'm watching similar genre movies, gathering information, brainstorming plots, lining up my editors and those people who will help me create my product. I'm creating something for the first time, and I'm hyper alert to stories around me that could build a better plot. I dream about characters. I'm releasing stress hormones like cortisol, adrenaline, and norepinephrine. There's tension and a bit of frustration in my struggle as I search for the plot. I don't want to sit down and write until I have more figured out.

2. **Release:** Finding a way to release your mind from what you're trying to do or create will help you get out of your own way. It's normal to struggle, but if we lean into it and use tools to help, we can lock into flow. (You might try the *Worry Time* idea on Day 18 to temporarily help you focus if thoughts of your loved one keep interfering with your success.)

You might feel like you're hitting a wall in this stage. Another suggestion is to meditate or take a walk in nature and ground yourself in the five senses. As you're walking, recite what you smell, taste, hear, see, and touch. Say each of these out loud, for example, "I smell burning leaves and hear them crunch beneath my feet. I taste the coffee from breakfast. I see green trees and brown branches, blue skies, and yellow daffodils."

We need to cut the ties to our struggle mindset, shift and pivot to something wholly different. This relieves us from the stress hormones that flood our system during the struggle phase.

3. **Flow:** In this phase, you go back to the task you were struggling with earlier and you're ready to go. You're

in your zone. You experience lateral thinking, pattern recognition, and near perfect decision-making. This is when you tackle a project and stay focused from the beginning until the end, without feeling any distractions or self-doubts.

For me, it's when I see a scene and write it all down without editing or stopping to change my mind. I write it as I see it and feel satisfied when it's complete.

It's important to note this phase can't exist independent of the two previous stages, and the next phase is equally important.

4. **Recovery:** This is the most important stage of the process. It's like sleep. We can't live without sleep. Flow drains our bodies of energy and taps into our reserves. It takes intentional rest to recover and regenerate more energy. The more you understand how to recover, the better you'll handle stress and the ability to get into flow again.

These four phases work together synergistically. Each specific sequence must be followed because flow can't exist without the other three. Each phase is important to the success of your dream.

Having a loved one with an SUD can still hack your flow, but if you're patient, deliberate, and intentional, you can get through the hiccups.

CLOSE YOUR GAP DAY 22: UNPACK YOUR CYCLE

Before we can enter the flow cycle, we must get out of the chaos cycle. Identifying our current chaos role can help us discover the best place to remove ourselves from the spinning wheel.

- Identify the relationships, environments, and circumstances that contribute to your chaos cycle. Journal these.

- Who, what, and when are outside factors robbing you of forward momentum on doing what you want to do?

- Determine your desire to change these factors and how you will change your role in the chaos.

- Can you recall a time when you were in flow? Describe that.

Notes from the All-Mighty Mom Tribe

Sandy

My Story

My son Ryan began drinking in high school. He had gone with "friends" somewhere we were not aware of, and he suffered a severe trauma that he was deeply upset and embarrassed about. When we noticed his changed behavior and asked what was wrong, he would not talk about it and insisted he was okay. He also suffered four concussions in high school—two of which were severe. He had bad headaches and used alcohol, spice, marijuana, and other substances to self-medicate.

We took him to doctors, but none were able to help him. He had his wisdom teeth pulled and was prescribed oxycodone, and he has since told us that when he took that first pill, his whole world was perfect, and he always wanted to feel that way. His personality changed, and he became very belligerent, rude, and disrespectful to us. He went to college and completed a bachelor's degree but mostly became addicted to alcohol and marijuana. We knew he was drinking too much, but with him living away from us, we did not know how bad his drinking was. He denied having any problem but got two DUIs during that time. He moved back in with us and could be charming when he wanted something but very ugly when he was drinking. He was an excellent liar, and I now see I believed way too many of his stories. He often got his way when asking for favors, and I now see I prolonged his recovery by not setting boundaries.

My husband saw through him but got angry and was able to stay out of it better than I did. We spent many hours talking to Ryan, trying to convince him that he could stop.

Of course, he couldn't, but we did not understand this. During this time, I was hyper aware anytime he was away from home. Every time the phone rang or my text dinged, I imagined the worst. I worried that he would be in an accident, overdose, or end up in jail. He spent some time sober because of court requirements, but he never "needed" to go to recovery. I worried that he would be sent to prison.

Tensions were high when he moved back in with us at twenty-four. He passed out in our front yard in February, and we had to call the ambulance. When he awoke, he was livid with us for having him taken to the hospital. He said he was fine and just needed to sleep it off. He told us that he wanted to die and had no reason to live. He went from being angry and defensive to sweet and trying to get his way.

I was easily manipulated. He drank alone in our basement and then his bedroom.

I would hear him running into things in the bathroom after I was in bed and couldn't sleep from worry.

I stopped going out with girlfriends and looked at my phone constantly in case Ryan needed anything.

I had lost myself and my life.

Fortunately, my husband and I were a team and handled boundary decisions together. We set them and stuck to them. We had set up driving contracts early on, and he lost the privilege of driving several times.

We finally decided we could not live this way any longer and gave Ryan a deadline to be out of our house. It was in the middle of the winter with COVID raging, but we were serious. He tried to find someone to live with but had no real friends. He got his third DUI.

When he returned from jail, we had a suitcase packed and told him that we would either take him to the homeless shelter or to a recovery program. He was finally ready to work on his issues and was in a recovery program for almost four months. He has moved to a sober living house, communicates with a sponsor, and attends AA, NA, or other support meetings most days of the week.

Desire to Change

I began to research community resources and was disappointed with all the barriers I ran into. The hospital and doctors were no help. Our community mental health center made appointments for counseling, but they were a month out or were rescheduled. I found Michelle Weidenbenner's "Moms Letting Go" Facebook group and learned of another mom who knew more about dealing with addicted loved ones, and both have helped me so much. I am now a member of Michelle's "All-Mighty Moms Tribe" and have learned so much about addiction and recovery, but most of all how to care for myself and grow into the mom God created me to be—filled with peace, joy, and happiness.

My Flow

Being in a state of flow is exciting and exhilarating! When I sew, I look at the challenge of a new project, study it, and begin cutting and sewing. With each step that works out, I get more energy. I lose track of time and do not want to eat. I just want to keep sewing. I can do this for hours.

DAY 23

Balance Bold Boundaries

*The only people who get upset about you setting boundaries
are the ones who were benefiting from you having none.*
—Unknown

Of all the subjects in recovery, moms struggle with boundaries the most. We don't know where we end, and our
children begin. After spending so much time as caretakers, we
need help severing the mommy tie and allowing our child to
develop his or her own identity, especially when they're sick
with addiction.

Some moms feel guilty when they learn how to set healthy
boundaries. Their boundaries feel wrong, mean, and disloyal
to their loved ones. If you're unfamiliar with healthy boundaries, setting them might feel awkward. The important thing
to remember is to express them in a loving tone without
explaining, making excuses, or feeling bad for giving them.

We want our children to develop a strong sense of self and believe they can do the work necessary to recover, but we can't carry their cross, take away their pain, or fix their problems. What we can do is strengthen our boundaries. If we can master our boundaries, we will have more time for the priorities that matter most.

Each of us has a different set of values, therefore our boundaries might look different from our friends or family members. What one person might tolerate another person might not.

I recommend working with a therapist. Many have developed unhealthy boundary patterns in childhood. Once we identify some of our weaknesses, we can begin the work of strengthening the boundaries that provide freedom. Healthy boundaries will cause your addicted loved ones to see you differently, respect you more, and allow them to learn from you. This change might take time, and a therapist can aid in the process.

How Will You Feel with Healthy Boundaries?

When you start trying out new boundaries, you might be tempted to make a bold stance. Others who don't share your values could feel shame or judged. They might see you as a boundary bully. This doesn't mean you should back down. Not everyone will understand. Be certain you've shared your boundary in love and keep taking care of yourself.

On the flip side, loosening your boundaries might make you feel overcommitted, which leads to burnout and breakdowns. Finding balance takes practice. Setting new boundaries will feel awkward in the beginning.

You'll know when you have established healthy boundaries because you'll feel calmer, more peaceful, empowered, confident, steady, joyful, and in control. Doesn't that sound desirable? You'll be able to listen to your loved one pour his frustrations out to you without lecturing, fixing, or getting angry.

What Do You Do with the Drama?

When our ALO calls to talk about the drama in his life, how someone stole his phone, someone at work snitched on him, or how his girlfriend or wife left him, it's important to pay attention to what happens inside of your body during these conversations.

If you can listen and ask open-ended questions, affirm their difficulty, and summarize their drama without feeling anxious or trying to solve their problem, then the BLESS Method using the PEACE Way to listen, and the Motivational Interviewing sections in Appendices A and B might help you listen with empathy.

On the other hand, if you feel yourself getting angry, starting to shake, or having trouble breathing every time they call or text, it's time to sort through feelings and set healthy boundaries. Your body is trying to tell you something.

When our body speaks, we need to listen. Let those feelings help you determine your bottom line regarding which dysfunctions you will and will not tolerate. If listening to the drama puts your mental, emotional, spiritual, or physical health at risk, then create pre-planned responses that will allow you to stay connected to your ALO without putting yourself in danger. Make sure they are something you can follow through with. Talk to a support partner about crafting these statements and give yourself permission to redirect or leave the conversation.

Your pre-planned responses may sound something like this: "It sounds like you're having a tough day. I'm sorry. I'll pray for you, but I have to cut this short. I'm in the middle of something." Or this: "Thank you for sharing your frustration with me, but I can't solve this problem for you. I'm confident you will find a solution." You could also say, "What will you do now? What are your options?" It will be difficult not to offer opinions, but the best boundaries include allowing your ALO to take responsibility. End each conversation with a calm affirmation: "I love you." "I believe in you." "You've got this."

If this boundary is new and your ALO expects you to come to his rescue, you might be tempted to call them back and recall your boundary. Find a support partner to help you through this temptation. Ask yourself, "Why do I feel the need to converse again?"

Most times the need stems from the desire to make sure your loved one understands and to calm your fears and anxiety regarding his well-being. Instead of making that call, take a walk in nature without your phone, listen to music, read scripture, or take a grandchild out for ice cream.

Our children will continue to push us to go past our boundaries. If you have time and your health isn't compromised, then drive them to work, take them to the doctor or to their probation appointment. You decide what you will and won't do. But keep in mind, each time they ask you to forgo your plans to care for them, your boundaries are being pushed.

When you're taking care of them, you're not taking care of you.

How Will You Know If Your Boundaries Are Weak?

If you feel overcommitted, taken advantage of, bullied, controlled, dominated, coerced, pushed, manipulated, or exploited, you're probably lacking boundaries. Your body's response might be fight (you get angry), flight (you run away), or freeze (you take the attack without having the energy to leave or fight). Weak boundaries can cause physical illness.

Here are some other symptoms of weak boundaries:

- You have difficulty speaking up.
- You give away too much time.
- You agree with someone even though inside you don't agree.
- You feel guilty taking time for yourself.
- You make too many sacrifices for others.
- You blow off your friends every time your ALO calls.
- You overshare details of your life.
- You feel guilty when your child doesn't feel happy.
- You attract people who try to control you.
- You fear what others think about you.
- You feel unappreciated.
- You fear abandonment.

Let these examples be warning signs. Pay attention to which ones you experience. Journal your feelings. Talk them over with your therapist.

My goal is for you to find your All-Mighty Mom status so you can achieve more—even if that more is peace.

If you don't have strong boundaries, don't feel bad. This takes time. I don't know one person who hasn't struggled with this topic at some point in her life. Sometimes our parents didn't set healthy boundaries, so we never got to see what they look like. It's never too late to start learning. You can teach your children and grandchildren.

What might happen when you set new boundaries?

- Your ALO will wonder what happened to you. This new you might make him angry, and he might scare you. Tell yourself he doesn't need to like you right now. It probably means you're setting a necessary boundary. If he likes you, it's probably because you're enabling his substance abuse.

- At first, it might feel funny to say no. But in time, you will find joy because you'll have more time for you and what you love to do.

- You'll attract other healthy friends to support. People like to be around confident people who don't complain.

- Eventually you'll feel more appreciated. It won't happen right away. But think about the last time someone did something for you. Didn't you appreciate them? When they quit taking you for granted, they'll become more appreciative.

- When we're not giving away all our time, we're able to sit with ourselves more and stay in touch with our needs.

- You'll be able to spend more time on yourself without guilt.

Studies about Complaining and Nagging

Excessive complaining or nagging can also be a sign you need to set boundaries. Plus, both have been shown to cause health issues. Listening to nagging or complaining for thirty minutes or more can cause damage to the part of your brain that handles problem-solving skills. In short, the habits of nagging and complaining are bad for us and for our loved ones.

Studies also show that complaining, like worry, increases the release of the stress hormone cortisol. Cortisol raises blood pressure and blood sugar, impairs the immune system, and can cause high cholesterol and diabetes.[31]

I challenge you to try not to complain or lecture for an entire day. If you catch yourself doing either, ask yourself a couple of questions:

Step 1. Am I allowing someone or something to infringe on my boundaries?

Step 2. Can I replace this action for something more constructive like reciting an affirming statement, learning a Bible verse, or finding gratitude?

Every time you start to complain or lecture, stop yourself and make a mark on a piece of paper. Redirect your actions using an example from Step 2. Tally your marks every day. See if you notice them lessening as you replace the negative habits with new habits.

As moms, we think it's our job to lecture, teach, and preach until our children get it right, even when they're adults. It's human nature; however, this approach doesn't work. When we scold our children into obedience, they feel shame. They withdraw and avoid us.

Every human craves connection and wants to feel loved. When meaningful connections are absent in a person's life, they may use addiction to fill the void.

It's important for us to find ways to stay connected to our addicted loved ones and maintain our healthy boundaries. This is where the difficulty lies. We hate seeing them destroy

> The opposite of addiction isn't sobriety. It's connection.
> **—Johann Hari**

their bodies and their lives, so we avoid them. Being on the receiving end of their rage makes us weary. They don't understand why we won't accept them into our homes, and they don't see their behavior as dysfunctional.

So how do we love our children, despite their addiction? Doesn't our love enable them?

Love means meeting them where they are while maintaining our boundaries. This objective is the most difficult task to master. Understanding the concept takes time, but you can learn if you're committed and intentional.

CLOSE YOUR GAP DAY 23: BALANCE BOLD BOUNDARIES

It's time for you to balance your boundaries.

1. What boundaries do you need to improve to achieve your Boon?

2. Which boundary weaknesses hack the most of your time? Take inventory.

3. Make a list of values and relationships that are a priority to you.

4. Make a list of what you can do for your loved one. Let them be responsible for finding help. Give yourself permission to say no. Sometimes reciting your boundaries out loud helps you practice staying strong and calm.

Notes from the All-Mighty Mom Tribe
Michelle

My Values

- Honesty
- Calm conversations
- Respect
- Honor my time
- Safety
- Sobriety

What I will do for my addicted loved one:

- Ask open-ended questions. Listen to what he's saying to affirm and summarize but only if my loved one is calm and sober.
- Pray with him.
- Empower him.
- Encourage him.
- Drive him to sober meetings and doctor appointments if he's in recovery and only if it's convenient for me. Encourage him to find his own rides first. If I agree to drive him or help him, he must be prompt, thankful, and respectful. If he violates these three rules, I have the choice to calmly drive off.
- Report abuse and/or neglect of grandchildren.

What I won't do for my addicted loved one:

- Give him money.
- Fix his car.

- Make excuses for him.
- Call in sick for him.
- Pay his rent.
- Allow his children to stay with him if he's using a controlled substance.

DAY 24

Recognize Your Neurochemicals

Whenever you want to achieve something,
keep your eyes open, concentrate and make sure
you know exactly what it is you want.
No one can hit their target with their eyes closed.

—Paulo Coelho

When you eat a piece of chocolate or have your coffee or tea in the morning, don't you feel energized? That's because your brain remembers this feel-good reaction and motivates us to seek more.

People are literally killing themselves using drugs or alcohol to find the perfect feel-good experience. Some want to relax, sleep better, think clearer, or get into their zone where they can forget their trauma or numb their pain. They don't plan to fall into the addiction trap; they think they can quit, until they can't.

When my son hurt his back and the doctor prescribed opioids, he discovered his productivity increased. He achieved hyper-focus and increased stamina on his job. Brain science confirms the first time our addicted children use drugs or alcohol, they have such an awesome experience, they want to try it again. The drugs trigger the pleasure center of our brains.

Alcohol and drugs overstimulate the reward circuit of the brain, the limbic system, which motivates people to use again. The brain remembers the positive feelings associated with the substance and motivates the person to use the drug again and again.

After repeated use, however, the brain adjusts to the increased dopamine signal. As a result, the ability to feel pleasure is reduced. The high the person once experienced no longer works. Soon the person needs drugs to feel normal. The more they use, they begin to feel lifeless, depressed, and unable to enjoy things that once brought them pleasure.[32]

This is where the disease takes over and makes it impossible to stop without severe physical consequences.

Flow

What if I told you that you could experience a similar high naturally, without using any substances or experiencing the negative consequences in your brain or body? You can—with flow.

God equipped our brains with everything we need to get into flow. The trick is to persevere in the struggle stage. This takes commitment and concentration.

So many people lose patience. They want immediate gratification, which might increase the appeal of substances. But we find joy when we wait for our reward and when we struggle through the pain.

Step Toward the Struggle

The enemy wants to abort your Boon. He comes to steal, kill, and destroy all God created you to be. He'll remind you of your failures and shame and trick you into wanting to quit. He knows how to seep into the crevices of your weak spots and place doubt in your mind. He'll make you believe you're not worth it, that you're a quitter, undereducated, incompetent, too poor, and the wrong person for this assignment. He'll try to convince you you're not strong enough, you don't have the time, or don't know the right people to succeed.

> There is joy at the end of every struggle we face. But you can never cross over and get there with the boats of complains. Complainer is only an explainer of pain! Take action!
>
> **—Israelmore Ayivor**

He is wrong! Decide right now to flick him off your shoulder. You can be everything God called you to be. When you realize the enemy inside your head is wrong, you begin to silence your inner critic. Once you do, you will find flow, that sweet spot that propels you toward achieving what you were called to create. Finding flow will allow your addicted loved one to see hope in you and want flow too.

Flow offers at least five benefits (see chart below) to motivate you by stimulating natural chemicals in your brain. Maybe these are heaven's gifts to help you achieve your Boon.

This chart from *Unhackable* by Kary Oberbrunner (page 204) demonstrates how the authentic chemicals produced by flow benefit us. Notice how one drug mirrors a feeling created by flow but with greater risks. It's worth noting the similarities because it helps us see how powerful flow can be and explains why so many people want to experience it the easy way, by consuming a drug.

AUTHENTIC	ARTIFICIAL	*BENEFIT*
NOREPINEPHRINE	Speed	increases heart rate, emotional control, attention
DOPAMINE	Cocaine	superhuman focus, pattern recognition, skill-enhacing abilities
ENDORPHINS	Heroin Oxycontin	withstand discomfort
ANANDAMIDE	Marijuana	augments lateral thinking, link contrasting ideas together
SEROTONIN	Antidepressants	stay on task in spite of pain

Moms Can Be Addicted Too

Moms can become addicted to the chaos and stress of living with an addicted loved one. If we grew up in a stressful and chaotic environment or experienced emotional abandonment, we may search for dopamine in places other than healthy relationships.

The pattern that almost consistently plays out in children and adults who have insecure attachments or an attachment disorder is the need to create excitement when things are calm and stable. This provides the dopamine release needed to feel alive and feel life has meaning and purpose.[33]

When dopamine levels dip, we feel a craving or a strong urge to engage in pleasurable activities, thus motivating us to repeat that activity. In this case it's our child's chaos or drama. Some moms think they want a calm and peaceful life, but when things become calm or peaceful, they're bored. They will think, *Why am I sad he's in recovery? Why do I have this empty feeling?*

Brains are complicated, and many adverse childhood experiences make it even more puzzling. The important thing to remember is the importance of our recovery for our children's sake. Studying family patterns and genograms (Day 22) can help us learn more about how we're wired and how to identify our blind spots.

If you catch yourself thinking about your child, your spouse, or your other children before yourself, and feeling restless when things are calm, it could be a sign that you have a need for excitement or chaos.

What if you could redirect your focus to creating your Boon? Would that bring the excitement you chase?

Triangulation

When things are chaotic with your ALO, who do you talk to? Do you reach out to your other children and share your frustrations? If so, you're not alone. Many moms talk to their healthy daughters and sons about their addicted children. It's easier to feel safe with family members. We don't want to share the nitty-gritty details with an outsider.

Unfortunately, bringing your other children into the chaos can put pressure on them. They might want to protect you from their sibling or become angry because of the addicted loved one's behavior or lack of respect. That child might not understand addiction or what motivates a person to use. This could cause a separation between siblings. Plus, your ALO will feel shame and rejection when he discovers family members are talking behind his back.

It's always better to talk to a professional or a private support group about issues involving your addicted loved one. These people have a detached, professional view. Additionally, bringing a third person into your relationship with your ALO could be beneficial if this person is a therapist, someone trained in mediating disagreements. A good, licensed counselor is able to see the situation from both perspectives, and if chosen correctly, could provide validation, affirmation, and empathy—those ingredients necessary for you to heal.

CLOSE YOUR GAP DAY 24: RECOGNIZE YOUR NEUROCHEMICALS

 How would you like to experience flow right now? Once you feel the power, you'll want to add it to your day more often. You will feel closer to God and experience His influence in your life. Follow the steps below:

1. Turn off distractions.
2. Get a pair of headphones and turn up the sound.
3. Prepare to be completely focused for five minutes.
4. Play *Synchronicity* on YouTube on full screen: bit. ly/SynchronicityMusic. (Or find your own favorite instrumental inspirational music).
5. Do nothing but watch the video.
6. Choose to let your mind go as you watch the video and listen to the music.
7. Afterward, write whatever comes to your mind in the space below. If you need silence, write in silence. If you'd like to listen to your song again while you write, then play it again. Don't edit. There are no wrong words. Flick your inner critic and the enemy off your shoulders.

My Micro Flow Session

_____

_____

_____

_____

_____

_____

_____

_____

_____

_____

_____

_____

_____

_____

_____

_____

_____

_____

_____

_____

_____

_____

Notes from the All-Mighty Mom Tribe

Lily

My thoughts immediately go to my goal for this year—to get the ball rolling on acquiring a solar farm for my mom on the ranch. This is her dream and mine—to make the ranch self-sufficient and fruitful—which is difficult in New Mexico, which has been in drought conditions for years.

The goal is to lease land to solar farm companies. The projected lease revenue could be $100,000 per year, which would make the ranch self-sufficient instead of the "money pit" that my husband imagines.

It would also give my recovering son a managerial position on the ranch, which he says he wants. It would provide him with the income to make much needed improvements on the ranch as well as paying for living expenses.

I envision the ranch house being updated—electrical systems, plumbing, HVAC, water supply, laundry, bathrooms, flooring, and eventually corrals, barns, and other animal pens.

I started to think about researching solar farm companies in the county where the ranch is situated and how to contact them.

I also have asked my recovering son if he would like to take part in the research and contacting of these companies, and he's going to help.

Ultimately that would give him purpose, a feeling of success if he is able to generate progress in moving toward this goal.

I believe that a one-year goal is reasonable for achieving this project goal.

Of course, the reality of developing the solar farm is several years from the initial leasing-to-completion of the placement and functionality of the solar farm itself. But one year to get the ball rolling is reasonable.

So, tomorrow I begin my research to make the family ranch sustainable and perhaps provide my son with purpose and a future at a place that has always been his refuge.

DAY 25

Understand Your Triggers

*The secret to change is to focus all your energy
not on fighting the old, but on building the new.*

—Socrates

We've mentioned our ALO's triggers, but did you know moms have triggers too? Our loved ones can trigger our temper, sympathy, guilt, shame, and pity. It seems they know us better than we know ourselves. They know how to manipulate us to get what they want, and most of us don't realize it or know it's happening. Our children aren't intentionally mean; they simply know what they must do to get what they want. If criticizing us elicits a weakness in our resolve, our children will poke at that hot stick all day until they get what they want: money, a place to stay, a car, a ride to a friend's house.

Only after celebrating two years in recovery could my son admit this fact. He said, "Addicts know how to get what they want." The diseased brain tricks them into believing their survival depends on using a controlled substance, so they will do whatever it takes to get what they need. We would do the same if we had to fight for food and water to survive. It's basic human nature.

Understanding and taking time to notice family patterns is important. Discovering our triggers can help us change. If we're oblivious to how our children manipulate us, we'll never embrace our goals. We'll be stuck in the hamster wheel of helping our child in the wrong way, taking responsibility for their actions instead of allowing them to grow from their mistakes, delaying their recovery and removing their motivation to change.

What can you do to find your triggers, understand them, and change your responses? Start with these tips:

Don't reply to anger with anger. Learn how to respond calmly. Reacting is an impulsive event, whereas, responding is thought out and controlled. One way to do this is not to take their manipulations personally. Once we understand the drugs or alcohol drive them, we can feel more comfortable saying no and take their criticism. If our ALO is mad at us, we're probably setting good boundaries. If they're happy with us, then we're probably taking the responsibility of their actions instead of allowing them to be responsible.

Journal. Each time you're triggered, journal and date the event. Record your feelings and how your responded or reacted.

Look for patterns. Review your journal every two weeks. What patterns do you notice? Do you give in to your child's demands or wishes when you pity him? Which emotion do you feel when you're triggered? Hurt? Pain? Guilt? Do you feel like you're responsible for your child's poor mental health or addiction?

Talk to a therapist. Tell her you're working to identify your triggers so you can overcome them. You might need to accept your role in your child's pain, ask for forgiveness, and/or give yourself grace. There might be trauma from your past you have to overcome. Don't ignore the importance of your mental health.

Join a support group. The right support group should give you the opportunity to share your frustrations and feel understood and heard. Ask the attendees to be your truth-tellers. Do they see patterns in your relationship with your addicted loved one that you don't see? This requires thick skin. Try not to react to what others share with you. Instead, listen and take time to process this information.

Roles We Play

When the chaos of addiction ensues, every person in the family takes on a role, like puppets on strings. Not until we do the work can we see where we fit. I listed a few of those roles below. See if you recognize yourself. I've played several. Ask your support group or other family members to identify which roles they've seen you play.

- **Policewoman.** She manages everything for the addicted loved one. She gets him up in the morning, keeps his calendar, and reminds him of events. The policewoman mom makes sure he's going to support meetings and probation appointments and administers drug tests. She polices who he's with and for how long. She bases her whole existence on keeping track of her ALO.

- **Lecture Queen.** This person lectures after every chaotic incident, confident her child learned his lesson. He discovers nodding in agreement to her sermon will get him what he wants.

- **Needer**. This person loves to feel needed. She might help even if no one asks.

- **Rescuer.** This mom believes jail is no place for her child because he's not like the others. She puts the safety net out every time her child gets in trouble and lets him land softly.

- **Dreamer.** This person believes what she wants to believe. She thinks her child is awesome and can't see the manipulation. She might have a spouse who sees things more clearly. These two perspectives often battle, causing more family dissonance and drama.

- **Shunner.** This person is angry and ashamed of her loved one. She's disowned him and won't talk to him.

- **Pushover.** This person loves everyone and aims to please. She wants the world to like her.

This list gives just a few examples of the roles we play. It's not intended to make you feel guilty. Hopefully, this list will help you evaluate your place in the relationship with your ALO and give you insight to understand and improve that relationship by abandoning your role. Because as often as our trigger sends us into our role, playing our role also feeds our triggers.

Leaving behind your role playing may increase the chaos for a short time. When we stop playing our role, our ALO can no longer rely on us to cover for them. They'll continue trying to manipulate until our actions convince them the scenario has changed. But this step in becoming unhackable will not only help us, but it will also ultimately be good for our ALO. Only when the pain of using a substance is worse than the pain of not using the substance will a person be motivated to change.

Good Triggers Keep Us in Flow

Most think of triggers as a bad thing, but there are positive triggers, too, ones that help us stay in flow. Understanding how positive triggers help us achieve optimal focus on whatever we're trying to accomplish, even on bad days, will help us cope better with our negative triggers. Here are five internal positive flow triggers:

The Deep Now

To experience flow, you must be in the present.

In the now, we can't see what happened in the past or worry about the future. Experts call this the Deep or Elongated Now. When we remain in the present, we stay away from switch-tasking. We embrace the acute pain and live from the gift of the present. Isn't it liberating to know it's okay, and healthy, to stop multitasking? I hereby declare you can stop multitasking from this moment on. You can live in the now, completing one task at a time.

If you find yourself slipping into the past or worrying about tomorrow, identify the emotion you're feeling and do an internet search for that word in the Bible. Find the verse that encompasses your emotion and ask God to release you from that trigger. Pray for a calm resolve.

A Defined Deadline

When we define our deadline, output is no longer optional.

Perhaps you've said, "Someday I'm going to _____." In this step, we define our someday. A deadline will make your Boon come alive. How many times have you heard, "I'm going to write a book," "I'm going to take a course," or "I should go back to college?"

You are different. You are a mom who wants to heal and accomplish your dream. Your output is no longer optional.

As we said on Day 13, a deadline isn't enough, though. Have you created urgency for your boom by setting a penalty for missing your deadline? Urgency will get you moving in full force. You're reading this book because you want to get well and focus on your dreams. You're not as young as you were, so if you want to leave a legacy, the time is now.

Authentic Ownership

Participation is mandatory, and you influence the outcome.

If you don't believe you and your contribution to building the Kingdom matter, then you're already out of flow. As you enforce the boundaries you've created and give up the role playing, you begin to take ownership of the real you. You decide how you will participate in the circus your ALO has created. Additionally, those boundaries transfer ownership of the problem back to the person to whom it belongs. When we take responsibility for our own actions and expect the same of our children, we create authentic ownership. This, in turn, creates confidence. We begin to see the importance of our mission. Our child may accuse us of arrogance at first, but when the outcome begins to blossom, they may decide they want authentic ownership too.

Real Risk

There's a personal cost for failing.

What is that cost for you? A pastor's risk might be that his congregation will leave the church and stray from God. A surgeon risks his patients' lives.

Addiction is a spiritual battle, and part of our fight is to overcome the enemy. We need help to fight. The risk of going it alone reminds me of a soldier going rogue. This realization should send us to counselors, therapists, support groups, and our knees.

Additionally, you and I risk our health. If we don't focus on our wellness, we'll be forced to focus on our illness. If our health suffers, we lose the ability to champion our Boon.

When we understand the true cost, our focus will change. Defining the real risk motivates us to stay true to our goal.

Rich Rewards

Our why gives us purpose.

I do this work because our children matter. I've been called by God to use my gifts and bring purpose to my pain. God never intended for the enemy to win. It motivates me to do my share to fight. How others view addiction and heal makes a difference. Bringing purpose to our pain helps us heal.

When I receive mail from moms telling me how much they've learned from me, healed, or thought they were alone until they found our group, my heart swells. The knowledge I'm doing something helpful for others is rewarding. It becomes an internal trigger, a motivator. Other moms who help in their community have told me that since they can't do anything for their incarcerated or addicted child, helping others gives them purpose. I pray you can find that too.

Experiencing flow is an internal goal, but it can help you achieve external goals like comfort, money, power, and fame. You can't have an internal goal without an external one. They are dependent upon each other. Kary Oberbrunner calls this the Boon Circle© in *Unhackable* (page 211).

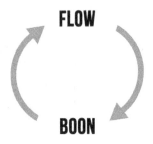

FLOW

BOON

External Flow Triggers

A Clear Goal

This is a big why combined with a big win. Why do you want to accomplish your goal or achieve your Boon? What's driving you?

Maybe you want to take an art class because it sounds peaceful and relaxing, but the thought of doing something new is intimidating. To help motivate you, imagine the reward. You could make new friends, discover a hidden a talent, or get lost in the process and find joy.

We can't predict the future of taking that class, but if you're excited about an art class, that's all that matters. If your why is important enough, it will carry you through. When your why is important, you will be motivated to accomplish it.

Consider Thomas Edison. He conducted numerous experiments before he invented the incandescent light bulb, and while working on a new type of battery with storage, a journalist visited.

> This [the research] had been going on more than five months, seven days a week, when I was called down to the laboratory to see him [Edison]. I found him at a bench about three feet wide and twelve feet long, on which there were hundreds of little test cells that had been made up by his corps of chemists and experimenters. I then learned that he had thus made over nine thousand experiments in trying to devise this new type of storage battery but had not produced a single thing that promised to solve the question. In view of this immense amount of thought and labor, my sympathy got the better of my judgment, and I said: "Isn't it a shame that with the tremendous amount of work you have done you haven't been able to get any results?"

Edison turned on me like a flash, and with a smile replied: "Results! Why, man, I have gotten lots of results! I know several thousand things that won't work!"[34]

Mercifully, Edison understood the laws of nature and the importance of perseverance—he integrated the feedback from each of those *failures*, changing one part of each experiment until he found the desired outcome.

> If you've always done what you've always done—you'll always get what you've got.
> —**Jessie Potter**

Here's my point. Though different than mine, your Boon is just as important. It is vital that we find ways to accomplish our Boons, and knowing our why helps.

Unpredictability

Neuroplasticity is the byproduct of new pathways.

Learning something new or participating in unfamiliar experiences causes your neural circuits to alter your brain. Neurons communicate with one another through special junctions called synapses. Repeated exposure causes these specific circuits to fire again and again. The stronger these synaptic connections become, the more your brain is rewired.[35] Understanding the unpredictability of new things can improve, my brain motivates me. I hope it motivates you too.

Feedback Loops

Truth-tellers fast-track flow.

Your art instructor points to your drawing and says, "Look at the angle of this object. Do you see how it's a bit off?" She then erases one of your lines and draws a new one. Instantly, you see the difference. You know she's guiding you.

We need external feedback, people willing to speak truth that will make us better. But to use it for flow, we must be willing to listen. You can find truth-tellers in support groups and places like the All-Mighty Moms Tribe. Accepting wisdom from people who've been on this journey as well as professionals can help us improve and achieve our Boon.

A Balanced Challenge to Competence Ratio

A perfect blend means I'll be perfectly present.

Some days I want to quit. I like the challenge, and my heart lies with my Boon, but when I have too much on my plate and I feel like I might snap, it's not a good day. To persevere, we need the perfect blend of stretching and achieving, pushing and resting. If the challenge is too difficult, or we push beyond our own competence, we will give up. To stay in flow, we must find that balance. Only you know what that balance is for you and your life.

CLOSE YOUR GAP DAY 25: UNDERSTAND YOUR TRIGGERS

Flow Trigger Assessment

For each question, circle the response that closest reflects your experience.

1. **The Deep Now:** When I focus on tasks, I don't think about my ALO or his problems.

   Never   Almost Never   Often   Almost Always   Always

2. **Defined Deadlines:** I have clearly defined deadlines with my ALO.

   Never   Almost Never   Often   Almost Always   Always

3. **Authentic Ownership:** I take responsibility for my flow and my Boon and expect my ALO to take ownership of his problems.

Never Almost Never Often Almost Always Always

4. **Real Risk:** I understand the risk to my own health and Boon if I continue to put my ALO's chaos first and set my priorities accordingly.

Never Almost Never Often Almost Always Always

5. **Rich Rewards:** I experience flow states, those moments where I'm in my zone, that place where nothing or no one hacks my productivity. These flow states integrate with my life, goals, and purpose so I reach my goals or Boon.

Never Almost Never Often Almost Always Always

6. **Clear Goal:** I have a big why combined with a big win. My happiness is not tied to my ALO's happiness. That's why I do what I do.

Never Almost Never Often Almost Always Always

7. **Unpredictability:** My brain experiences large amounts of neuroplasticity. I can rebound quickly if my ALO is using and/or in jail or homeless.

Never Almost Never Often Almost Always Always

8. **Feedback Loops:** I have truth-tellers and support groups to help me stay calm and healthy. I listen to the truth-tellers who tell me when I'm enabling, shaming, lecturing, or not listening.

Never Almost Never Often Almost Always Always

9. **Challenge to Competence Ratio:** My life is a perfect balance of high challenge and high skills. I can keep my emotions calm and respond to my ALO without reacting with high emotions, so I can stay focused on my personal growth.

Never   Almost Never   Often   Almost Always   Always

Flow Trigger Scoring

Count the number of answers above in each of the five categories and write that number in the respective blank below:

Never: ___ x 1 = ___
Almost Never: ___ x 2 = ___
Often: ___ x 3 = ___
Almost Always: ___ x 4 = ___
Always: ___ x 5 = ___
TOTAL: _____

Multiply each number you wrote by the number to the right.

Total all five numbers from the evaluation above and reference the Flow Trigger Key below:

- 1–9: My life contains little to no flow. I am under-performing. I rarely accomplish things. And I don't feel satisfied.

- 10–18: I have experienced flow a few times. When I did, I felt great, but my life doesn't contain enough positive triggers to reproduce it on a regular basis. I have more negative triggers that get in my way.

- 19–27: I experience flow sometimes. My life contains some of the required positive triggers to help me get into flow. I feel great about 50 percent of the time.
- 28–36: I often experience flow, certainly more times than not. My life contains many flow triggers, and I often feel my best and do my best.
- 37–45: My life is organized around positive flow and leaning on God to overcome my negative triggers. I experience Optimal Human Performance daily, and because of this, I do my best and feel my best.

My Flow Trigger Plan

To get more flow, I will implement the nine flow triggers into my life taking the following clear and specific actions:

_____

_____

_____

_____

_____

_____

_____

_____

_____

_____

_____

_____

Notes from the All-Mighty Mom Tribe
Michelle

My score was a thirty-seven today. When I first took this assessment, it was ten points lower. I have noticed that when I'm worried about whether my son has had a recurrence, I don't stay in that space for long. I sit with my emotions and ask myself three questions:

1. Do I know what I'm thinking to be true?
2. Do I know that it's absolutely true?
3. Who would I be without these thoughts?

I realized that most of my thoughts are fears that never come true. Feelings aren't facts. Yes, it helps that my son is in recovery, but there will always be something to worry about. I'm going to choose to live my life and create my legacy because that's the only life I can control. But leaning into my faith is a huge part of my letting go.

***

Lucretia

Self-care matters! If you don't take care of your wellness, you will be forced to take care of your illness.

Our deepest pain can bring our greatest rewards. In other words, there is pain in the process. We learn from pain.

As moms, we are continually letting go of something or someone during our lives. It's painful to let go. How do we cope? It's scary to let go and let God work. We must get out of the way for God to work. It's okay to let go and have joy in our lives, but it takes work when there is chaos around us.

My triggers come from re-experiencing trauma. Different types of memories can stir my emotions: anger, anxiety, loneliness, stress, grief, pain, sadness, and more. Your triggers might vary from mine, but I think moms share a lot of the same ones.

There was a time when my brain was so consumed with my son's addiction I was living on raw emotions and nerves. My emotional triggers were coming more and more often, and I wasn't listening to my body. My health and my daily life was hacked.

I started having seizures. At first, I thought they were from low blood sugar, but blood tests revealed my blood sugar was normal. Stress was causing me to shake and have blackouts.

I needed a plan. I needed to listen to my mind and body, so I started journaling about what events led up to my triggers—what made them happen and how I felt afterward.

The negative behavior from my son had to stop affecting me this way. Enough was enough! I couldn't continue living this way. That's when I realized I wanted him to heal more than he did.

First, I wrote down my boundaries—what I would do and what I wouldn't do. I chose to be strong, focus on Jesus, and let Him work in my life.

I renewed my mind by studying Romans 12:2. Another verse that spoke to me was Philippians 4:6 (NIV): "Do not be anxious about anything, but in every situation, by prayer and petition, with thanksgiving, present your requests to God."

Next, I needed prayer warriors and a support group because my family was tired of hearing about the chaos. I craved other moms who understood what I was going through. That's when I found the All-Mighty Mom Tribe.

My Role: Many times, I was the policewoman and the lecture queen. I thought if I could control my son's life, then my life would be less stressful.

When my son lost another job or slept all day then was up all night, my lectures would begin again. I didn't understand the diseased brain and thought he would simply quit if I could just get through to him. He would want to make the right adult decisions and not hurt me. My lectures didn't work.

I needed to gain knowledge about addictive behaviors. Once I studied more about addiction, I realized why my lectures didn't help me or my son. I took ownership of my mental and physical health.

My addicted son, who is a grown man, had to take ownership of his own life.

Yes, it's tough growing up! But we all do. When I stopped lecturing and helping in the wrong ways, change started happening in me and in my son too.

There were risks, but I did it scared. I knew God would be with me. He promised He would never leave me or forsake me. I had to cling to this and keep taking the next steps. **I kept telling myself that God loves him more than I do**.

This became my mantra. I repeated this to myself every day, some days many times.

Stressful situations, like when my son was homeless for months and in prison, or when the baby momma was addicted and arrested, and the abandoned grandchild needed to be taken care of, took more intentional focus.

There were times when the stress caused more triggers, which led to more seizures. I would be wiped out for several days afterwards with headaches, no energy, brain fog, and mental fatigue.

There is no warning when this happens, so it's scary.

For the last several years, I have been decreasing my stress, making healing choices, and not letting the enemy stress me out.

Learning about how stress triggers my brain and causes my seizures is helping me learn new coping skills.

I am working on rewiring my brain with knowledge, scriptures, music, exercise, nature, and taking time for me.

This addictive disease is a spiritual battle, and as moms, we must battle it on our knees in prayer.

You may respond differently to your triggers than me, but leaning into your emotions and understanding why you are triggered will help you heal and change.

We can't go back and relive the past, but we can learn from it. We must move forward to take the next right step.

DAY 26

Assess Your Growth

*What you do makes a difference, and you have to decide
what kind of difference you want to make.*

—Jane Goodall

One of the moms in our Moms Letting Go group, Beth Marie, lost her son, Joshua, to an overdose. We were devastated for her. We all thought, *This could be my child.*

She said, "I loved him with all my heart. No regrets . . . and when they sneak in, I remember God was and is in control." She says, "Step back, Satan. You might think you won Josh, but you didn't. Yes, he died from those evil drugs, but he knew and lived for the Lord! He is in heaven, and his death will bring about great things, just like his life did. I'm clinging to this thought to survive."

Beth Marie remains active in our group and finds comfort in encouraging moms and sharing her story.

In 2011 and 2012, she underwent two extensive back surgeries. They put a twelve-inch rod in her back, eight cages to support her discs, and lots of nuts and bolts. She said, "I'm a scrap metal collector's dream."

Beth Marie was in constant pain, unable to stand, sit, or lie down. To cope, she rolled paper beads by taking tiny strips of paper, rolling them around a skewer, and shaping them into a bead. She used them to make bracelets, necklaces, and bookmarks. It was tedious work, but her hands were the only things that were still useful.

She sat for hours at the dining room table so she could forget her physical pain. As she rolled, she prayed. When she created a necklace for her aunt, for instance, she prayed and recalled times they spent together. She called this flow. In this flow state, she never had pain.

Eventually, her bead rolling turned into a side business that served her well in that painful season.

She said, "In pain management class, they call this mentally putting your pain on the back burner. The professionals referred to physical pain, but we can do this with our mental pain, anguish, and worry too. It's healthy!"

Why am I sharing Beth Marie's story? Because it gives us an example of how we intentionally move past our pain and bring value to others. Physical, emotional, spiritual, or relational—no matter our state of pain—we can experience flow when we give it a purpose. I'm excited to see where God will lead Beth next in His tremendous plan.

Liminal Space

Liminal space is that uncomfortable space between where you are and where you want to be. It's when you're on the verge of something new, but you're not quite there yet. It's uncomfortable because we crave predictability, and liminal space isn't predictable.

Moms of addicted loved ones often get stuck in this space. Our lives are suspended between what our lives were like before our child had an SUD and what we think our lives will look like when our child is in recovery. If we knew for certain our children would recover, it would be easier to get through the havoc. But there are no guarantees.

If we stay in this liminal space, it can have harmful effects on our mental health. Instead, if we look at this space as an opportunity for transformation, we can intentionally seek change. But first, we must accept where we are and agree that we want to change.

If we look at Beth Marie's story and follow the hero's journey, her inciting incidents were back surgery in one story and Josh's death in another. Both events profoundly changed her life. She could have stayed stuck in liminal space, unwilling to move on, but she chose to move past her pain and transform into purpose.

You can do the same if you intentionally find your way and choose change.

Your Boon Ceremony

You're about to head into the Boon Ceremony, the final part of this program. In it, you'll have the chance to be brave and tell your truth with the whole Tribe listening. You're ready because you've grown the past twenty-five days. You should feel yourself getting stronger. You've been consuming the content and integrating it into your life. You've been barreling toward your Boon and becoming unhackable.

CLOSE YOUR GAP DAY 26: ASSESS YOUR GROWTH

It's time to assess your growth. Take some time today to look back over your story from Part One. Consider your level of hope before starting this journey and evaluate how your focus has changed over the past few weeks.

- How have you grown since the beginning of this book?
- What have you learned about your addicted love?
- Big or small, how has your thinking changed?
- What is your biggest takeaway from this book so far?
- What actions will you take and apply after reading this book?

Notes from the All-Mighty Mom Tribe

Brooke

Since the beginning of the book process, I have become calm and grounded on most days.

I understand that my grown son's actions are not under my dominion. I would love to make all the hard things (consequences) disappear, but I can't. So, I have put efforts toward making my life more fulfilling and helping those who truly want assistance.

I have learned my son suffers greatly with a substance use disorder. He is the target of societal exasperation and misunderstanding. I do not want to contribute to the ridicule. He is my child, and I love him. While I cannot enable, I also cannot hate. The line is tricky, but he's worth trying to find the right balance.

Understanding addiction and its insatiable grip on the human mind and emotions has been transformative to my perception of my son.

My biggest takeaway has been realizing my life matters too. My identity is more than being a mother and grandmother.

I have taken the action of changing jobs and career paths. I am in a happier place at work, and I'm making a living wage for the first time. I am also happy to have the chance to share a bit of my story in this book. I have made weekly hot yoga and tai chi part of a self-care practice that is improving my balance and confidence.

PART FIVE

The Boon Ceremony

DAY 27

Clarify Your Boon

*Try not to become a man of success but
rather try to become a man of value.*

—Albert Einstein

Welcome to the first day in the last section of *Unhackable*.
You've come a long way. Many moms will never make it
to this day, but you did. This is where you see how far you've
come. We're going to recap previous days to help you see your
progress on this journey, and I'm hopeful your Boon is clearer.

When I wrote my seven-step book, *Moms Letting Go
Without Giving Up*, I knew I wanted to help moms of addicted
loved ones, but I didn't have all the details spelled out. I still
don't. I took imperfect action and started where I was with
what I knew and what I had. Since then, the clarity of my
Boon and my leadership skills have grown. If I hadn't believed
God walked with me, I couldn't have kept going. Faith is a
huge reason I'm where I am today. I've walked through the
fog. Fortunately, today the path looks clearer, though some
days the fog still grows thick. I've discovered when I keep

walking, trusting, and praying for a clearer vision along my way, I gain clarity. God will guide me.

I learned many valuable lessons along the way, but two have really stuck with me. First, little steps lead to big payoffs, and next, it doesn't take as much time, money, and energy to bring value to others as I thought it would.

Don't Hack Yourself

Before we go any further, let's look at where you've been because it will motivate you to keep going. Here's a recap:

On Day Two, you picked your Boon. If you're like most moms, you weren't sure what your Boon was on that day. Maybe you left that day blank or chose peace for your Boon because you couldn't think past your need for peace. As you may have discovered, peace comes with unhackability. After we learn how to let go of the chaos, responding instead of reacting, we find we can do more. I pray that's where you are today: able to see in the fog, feeling the clouds lifting. Rewrite your Boon from Day Two or write an updated Boon based on all you've learned over the past twenty-six days.

_____

_____

_____

_____

On Day Five, you counted your cost. What fears did you have about achieving your Boon? Be honest. Rewrite those fears below. Do those fears still scare you? Why or why not? Record your feelings.

_____

_____

_____

_____

On Day Six, you claimed your promise. If we believe that our idea, or Boon, came from God, and He is working through us, we will feel more empowered to continue. Remember your why. Why does this work matter to you? What makes you passionate about achieving your Boon? What will it look like when you accomplish your Boon? Your job is to believe in yourself. I believe in you, but it's not enough. You must believe in you. Write your why from Day 6.

_____

_____

_____

_____

On Day Ten, you created your Boon road map. So often we want to know exactly what we're supposed to do in the next season of our lives, but that's not the way it works. We must take small steps in new directions, if they fit. New territory feels uncomfortable. The only way to learn something new is to step in and take imperfect action. We can't expect to know everything on the first day of the job. We gain clarity because we act. You did your best to create your Boon Sheet. Rewrite it here or update it to fit your updated Boon.

_____

_____

_____

_____

On Day Thirteen, you created your space. You established deadlines for your boundaries with your ALO and your boon. Creating a penalty for missing your deadline injects a serious dose of motivation. In the Tribe, I promised to give away three twenty-five-dollar Amazon gift cards if I didn't finish this book by September. I set a deadline and created urgency with a penalty. I'll be out seventy-five dollars. Today, revisit or rewrite your Boon Contract.

_____

_____

_____

On Day Twenty-One, you acknowledged your grief. We've all lost something precious. It's important to accept that and move through the stages of grief so we can journey through the stages of recovery. You discovered it was time to get out of your way, throw away your self-limiting beliefs, and write your Boon Poem. Rewrite it here.

_____

_____

_____

_____

CLOSE YOUR GAP DAY 27: CLARIFY YOUR BOON

Now that you've finished your recap, you can see how far you've come. Are you happy with your progress? If so, what stands out the most to you? Has your Boon grown, changed, or expanded?

_____

_____

_____

_____

Journaling is a valuable tool to help us see our progress. Looking back, we can connect the dots. This allows us to remember the details and acknowledge the pain. Journaling our progress enables us to recognize our triggers and the places we get stuck. This Big-Picture view teaches us better ways to control our lives. When we notice problems and fears, we can prioritize our focus. It provides an opportunity to identify negative thought patterns, behaviors, places to improve, as well as positive self-talk.

Clarity is life changing. You know when to say yes and when to say no. Just like traveling to your dream destination, identifying your Boon map and the route to get there gives you so much focus you won't settle for anything less. Not to mention the energy you save on your journey.

With each step, you will move with clarity toward a generous income—whether monetary, relational, spiritual, physical, or emotional. You _will_ be rewarded for the work you've done.

Each time you feel hacked, come back to this chapter; use it to remember and refocus. You've worked hard to get here. It's time to start the celebration.

Notes from the All-Mighty Mom Tribe
Brooke

My Boon is to help people who do not have homes.

When my son with a substance use disorder (Micah) was a little boy, his heart broke for people without homes. When he was eight years old, we went to a Miami Heat basketball game. He had saved his allowance for weeks because he wanted to buy a jersey from the Heat Store. But as we were approaching the door of the arena, a homeless man approached our family asking for money. My husband and I were not carrying cash, so we apologized but continued walking toward the arena. Micah paused, opened his wallet, and gave all his money to the unhoused man.

We had no way of knowing Micah would be homeless one day as the result of his addictions.

Remembering the tenderness in Micah's little heart, and knowing that I cannot ease the burden of homelessness for Micah because he needs recovery, I decided to assist people without homes who want to change.

I am a Board member for PIVOT TN, an organization whose aim is to provide permanent housing solutions for those who do not have homes.

We are making inroads to help people in our community. The first step was to find overnight shelter for those sleeping outside. Through a cooperative effort with other nonprofits, we have purchased an overnight shelter and are working to get the building up to code so it can be used as a temporary solution.

I am happy with that progress.

What stands out most to me is the amount of work required to move a person, or an organization, forward. We have worked for two years, and we do not have any solutions in place. I see progress but certainly not perfection. I look forward to the fruits from all our labors!

My Boon has changed. PIVOT began in hopes of building tiny homes for those without houses. Then we saw the need for overnight shelter, especially in cold weather. As a result, our focus shifted to cooperating with other nonprofits so we could purchase a shelter. That's been purchased but isn't operational just yet.

Our long-term goal is still providing tiny homes for the homeless, but we've had to shift to more practical initial steps.

DAY 28

Craft Your Boon

Stay afraid, but do it anyway. What's important is the action.
You don't have to wait to be confident.
Just do it and eventually the confidence will follow.
—Carrie Fisher

S andy Swenson wasn't always a published author ministering to moms of addicted loved ones. She once lived life stuck in the addiction chaos like all of us. She slew many dragons before breaking free and starting her publishing journey. She experienced days of self-doubt. People stood in her way, but she stayed true to her voice. She found healing through her God-given gift of writing. Though she started writing for herself, Sandy found she could help moms like you in the process.

A Note from Sandy

I started writing at the suggestion of a friend as a place to put all the thoughts, fears, and mistakes I'd been carrying around for so long. She thought it might lighten my load so I could sleep at night and focus on the other people I love during the day. I needed a place to store all the things swirling around my head, heart, and life, a place I could return to when I needed to put together the pieces of the child-consuming addiction puzzle I was living—but I never did. It turned out just putting pen to paper brought unexpected healing.

I had never kept a journal, but I quickly filled about ten pages with rambling scribbles. These pages revealed patterns of thought, actions, and reactions I would have otherwise missed. They led me to change the way I responded to the disease. That's when I decided to write a book, the book I needed when I started my journey—all the truths, love, and power we moms have in fighting this horrible disease—including the truth that our love cannot fail, even if our child doesn't find recovery.

My son struggles with addiction, and it has changed every fiber of my being. I am much stronger than I ever thought possible. I'm more patient, less judgmental, and hopefully, much wiser. I have learned to recognize and focus on what I can change and control—me. And I've learned the power of acceptance, unconditional love, and honoring my child (not the addict), as well as the fact that helping other moms on this journey helps me heal too.

As mothers of children suffering with addiction, we battle a disease that oozes misunderstanding and shame. Alone and afraid, we try to do the right thing—even when we're not sure what that right thing is. We try to hold our families and ourselves together even when it feels like we're falling apart. We feel every pain our child feels, no matter the distance (in miles or years). We try to carry on, even when our heart is breaking. But as tired and tattered as we may be, like the deceptively delicate dandelion, we moms persevere.

Together, we travel a most unwanted, unanticipated, and unclear journey—a journey that lasts a lifetime. Whatever happens next may, or may not, follow a neat or hopeful path. So, we all need to find our inner dandelion, to take a closer look at things we don't want to look at—the things lurking around in this place where love and addiction meet—so we're as strong as we can be.

Whenever I sit down to write, I write as a mom, the mom of an addicted loved one and, specifically, the mom of a son—a mom who has begun her own recovery, though her son has not.

My writing comes from deep within this specific mix. The voice burbling up comes from the well of my own experience; however, I believe it reflects the heart and soul of every mother of an addicted loved one. I hope to help put words to your thoughts and feelings, to help you heal.

Recovery is a process we all share. It's not only for the health and well-being of our beloved addicts but also for the rest of our families—and ourselves. On the road to recovery, we pass through several stages—sometimes again and again, often all cattywampus, and always in our own good time.

When addiction takes root in our child, we may be completely unaware. But once we've heaved ourselves over the monstrous hurdle of realization, the recovery journey begins: We learn, we grow. We cry, we wilt. We learn the value of nurturing ourselves. We find strength, we bloom. And finally, like fields of frazzled flowers, we scatter seeds of truth and goodness, changing the dynamic of this place where love and addiction meet. One by one, and one after another, we are carried aloft by the hope, the help, and the beating hearts of other mothers who love a child suffering with addiction.

We may often feel fragile, but we are strong—and we are many.

We have the capacity to overpower the destruction that addiction spreads.

Before She Started

Before Sandy started writing, she didn't know who she would inspire or if she would make a difference. But that couldn't stop her; she didn't let fear get in the way. Based on the volume of her book sales, speaking events, followers, and the emails she receives, countless moms have been inspired.

She said, "I know my message has reached many tens of thousands of moms.

"I remember someone telling me very early on that I would be grateful for this journey, but I can emphatically state that is not true for me. This has been the worst thing I could ever imagine. And then some. I am grateful, however, for discovering the strong person tucked away inside this old gal—stronger than may have ever emerged without life's most difficult challenges.

"I was not a writer before I wrote my first book. I was not a public speaker, not a voice for anything. But my child's addiction changed everything. I am now an author and speaker; I have something to say.

"There are countless ways we can turn our pain into purpose. We just need to believe in ourselves and our gifts and dive in."

Pain into Purpose

Here is an excerpt from Sandy's book, *Tending Dandelions: Honest Meditations for Mothers with Addicted Children.*

> I'm learning to live without my child, but, like someone whose leg has been amputated, through force of habit I often reach for the place he once was. The pain I feel is not phantom. If I'm to survive, the void left behind must be filled with some goodness.

There's so much hurt in the world. Hurt is happening all around me, not only within me. There are other lost parents who are missing a lost child. And the children who are lost. There are lost souls who are hungry, lonely, or running on empty. I don't need to look very far to find ways to turn my pain into purpose. Ways to be constructive. Productive. Ways to help keep others from breaking, even as I mend my own self.

I can hold a hand, lend an ear, and watch over with care. For them. For me. But also, in honor of my child. Addiction has hacked my child from my life, but He will be with me every step of the way as I move forward.[36]

What about you? If you knew others were waiting for you to help them, what would you do? How would you use your God-given gifts to inspire others? What part of you was created to help others?

Sandy hears from moms almost every day. She also has a collection of dandelion gifts from moms who feel a connection with her. Do you remember the letter you wrote on Day 5 from a fictitious follower? What if one of your letters looked like the ones below from Sandy's followers?

I'm here to tell you this can happen to you because God created you for a purpose.

Real Letters from Fans

"Having someone I never met describe my world and my heart so accurately is an incredible gift and in a strange way, blindingly beautiful. I'm so sorry for your pain; I know it well. Please keep writing! Without question, it is helping many fellow travelers."

***

"I am speechless; you have just told my story. Thank you."

***

"This is beautiful and has deeply touched me and given me an aha moment of sorts! Thanks for what you do. We all must stand up, speak out, and destroy the stigma of addiction."

***

"I met you when you were speaking in Florida a few weeks ago, and you truly inspired me! I admire you so much because it is easy to be positive and detach when your child is in recovery. But you manage to do that when your son is not and continue to love and pray for his recovery while finding a place of serenity for yourself. I believe the journey of your family will help many families suffering from this disease."

***

"Thank you for openly sharing your experience with your son. It's because of your book that I'm alive today. I believe my strength to grieve my firstborn comes in part from you, Sandra. Had you not shared your journey, I'd be lost on mine."

***

"Sandy, if I think of one person that has made an enormous impact on other's lives, I think of you."

***

"Truly amazing how Sandy has put into words the deep suffering, heartache, resilience, and hope for many dealing with an

addicted child. She so eloquently shares her story with openness, honesty, and strength through her life's ups and downs from her son's disease of addiction, divorce, aging, elderly parents, uprooting, along with helping so many with her books."

CLOSE YOUR GAP DAY 28: CRAFT YOUR BOON

You'll always have naysayers and doubters trying to make you second guess what you want to do. Sometimes, your strongest resistance will come from the lies you believe about yourself. Confront those lies. What are they—no time, no skill set, no money?

- Journal the lies you believe.
- List the emotions that hold you back.
- Do an internet search for scripture about each of those emotions.
- Read the Bible.
- Find the verse that speaks to you most.
- Recite it out loud.

When we have faith, we believe we will find the time, skills, and finances. We stay in touch with our higher power. Having a relationship with God is key if we're going to understand our calling.

Today, as you craft your Boon, you'll have to decide which script to write—the one your lies want you to believe or the one you know you need to write.

Don't worry about the typos, misspellings, grammar problems, or sentence structure. Use your notes from the past month. Do what you need to do to get into flow. Don't edit. Just write what's in your heart, what you see yourself doing or building.

This will be called your Boon Speech. Try to keep it to five minutes. If you need inspiration, ask yourself these questions:

- What makes me angry?
- What causes me to cry?
- What brings me joy?
- What fuels my passion?

When you're passionate about a topic, you'll have the energy to implement your gifts.

Write Your Boon Speech

_____

_____

_____

_____

_____

_____

_____

_____

_____

Notes from the All-Mighty Mom Tribe
Michelle

My Boon Speech

Have you ever wondered why you were born? I mean, what's your purpose?

The two most important days of our lives are the day we were born and the day we discovered why.

Why were you born?

The million-dollar question. Was it to inspire someone? Was it to birth one of your children or all of your children?

Sometimes we spend our whole life trying to figure this out. I'm right there with you.

My why changed like the seasons, depending on where God was calling me.

Each time I wrote a book, I thought the book's "message" was my why.

Then my son and daughter-in-law became addicted to opioids and then heroin and then meth. While I was going through this chaos in my life, I couldn't figure out where I was supposed to be. Some days I couldn't breathe for fear they would die. Some days I felt their anger directed toward me, even though I had kept their children safe.

Other days, I searched for moms who also had addicted children because I didn't know what to do or what to say. I craved a mentor. I was sick with worry, anger, and frustration. Why couldn't they get their lives together?

Until one day, I realized that this was my calling. If not me, then who? Yes, God needed me to help other moms. I found my mentor. It was God.

But who was I? I certainly didn't have all the answers. All I knew was how to write a book, so I created a journal for moms to work through. To heal. To find self-care.

And that's where my purpose started.

Since that moment, I've created the book and video tutorials, courses, a podcast, and built a community, and now I know.

I want to empower one million moms of addicted loved ones to get into recovery by 2025.

What is recovery for the mom of an addicted loved one?

It's personal. It's not the same for each mother because we are all different. Each mom has a different Boon, but if I speak in generalities, I'd say recovery for these moms is to recapture their purpose and joy. In doing so, they will empower their addicted children. They will be the Chief Hope Builders, Hope Medics, who show the way, who help their children see the endless possibilities of living for a higher purpose and achieve their dream.

Through my leadership, and those moms who gather with me, we will ignite other Hope Medics worldwide. In doing this, we will unite moms to stop the stigma and bring addiction recovery solutions—evidence-based solutions—to everyone. We will love those people with a substance use disorder in jails and prisons and help them find their purpose and an alternative way to heal from their trauma and disease.

We will be the All-Mighty Moms creating a movement for addiction change.

Unhackable. Unstoppable. Fearless Warrior Moms.

DAY 29

Communicate Your Boon

People who are crazy enough to think they can change the world are the ones that do.

—Steve Jobs

Eight years ago, I published my first novel. My granddaughters were eight and three. I never could have predicted I would write this book about addiction and bring hope to moms. I knew my son and daughter-in-law had problems, but who didn't? I believed they'd work them out. I never thought they would become so sick they would almost die.

Back then I wouldn't have thought I'd be called by God to lead moms in a ministry, but here I am, more passionate about it than anything else in my life. This work matters, but I can't do it alone.

Thank you for being on my team, for wanting to recover so you can be the best version of yourself. You're an All-Mighty Mom, and today I'm celebrating you and the thousands of moms who have joined our efforts to recover.

The Boon Ceremony

Imagine standing in an auditorium filled with moms who understand your pain. They also have an addicted son or daughter. They've tried to help, seeing failures and successes along the way. They've lost sleep, money, and relationships because of addiction. Some have lost children to fentanyl poisoning.

Today, they're standing together holding hands, swaying, and singing worship songs.

These moms, like you, stepped into their recovery so they could journey on a path to help fight addiction using the gifts God has given them. Some moms want to work on finding a cure or stop the stigma and change the jail and prison sentencing for those with an SUD. Others want to start jail ministries or go back to school and become therapists. No two Boons look the same because every mom has a different story. But we understand each other.

Each one of these women boasts the title *All-Mighty Mom on Fire*. Each has a Boon to bring change to the addiction world.

In this imaginary auditorium, the music stops. One at a time, each mom walks to the front of the room. She shares her name, the name of her addicted loved one, and her Boon. Each has done the work to earn a spot on the stage of the Boon Ceremony. No Boon is too small. It's the baby steps that lead to a movement.

As each mom steps to the microphone, the room grows quiet again. Every person in the room knows the courage and perseverance it took to get to this moment. The stories inspire tears, and the hushed whispers of prayer sound like soft music accompanying each speaker. As the last mom finishes, applause thunders, some whistle, while others sob. The hair on your arms stands; you can feel the electricity in the room. Their inspiration makes you want to shout your plan.

One Important Detail

Before change can take place, we need to rally. You chose this book because you want to do something different; you read to change yourself and your community. Healing happens best in community. I want you in the room with other women declaring their Boon Speeches. Thank you for your desire to be part of something big. We can't change our addicted loved ones, but we can be part of stopping the cycle, serving in a place that will be the catalyst for change.

One person can make a difference, but a tribe of Mama Bears fighting with their dukes up, teeth bared, and voices loud can create a movement.

CLOSE YOUR GAP DAY 29: COMMUNICATE YOUR BOON

It's time to share your Boon. Communicating your Boon might be out of your comfort zone, but it may help to remember this: the message you share comes from God. It isn't about you; it's about God working through you. God counts on you to use your gifts in the building of the Kingdom. He doesn't care if you stutter or repeat yourself. He doesn't care if you aren't perfect.

Communicating your Boon will help curb your nervousness. When we take ourselves out of the equation and focus on serving others, we worry less about people judging. There's no wrong way to act. We take imperfect action and learn *on the grow*. Each time you say your Boon out loud, you will gain confidence. Your conviction will strengthen because others will encourage you. You'll start seeing signs of God opening doors. It's a powerful feeling, but remember, you might not recognize the open doors until you realize you walked through.

Your Boon has nothing to do with your loved one's recovery. It's intentional and attainable. Once you recapture your identity and find your purpose, you will be an *All-Mighty Mom on Fire*. I'm anxiously waiting to hear your Boon and help you share it with others so they can be inspired too.

I recommend you work this program in a group so you can celebrate with a huge Boon Ceremony. People who share their passion with others and find validation in their Boon help each other overcome self-limiting beliefs and leave a legacy. I want that for you.

Unhackable Boon Speech Process

Yesterday you wrote your speech. You dug deep into your feelings and squelched the lies. It's time to record your speech. Use your phone or your computer. Ask a friend to help. Then post your speech online—either on your Facebook profile, or in the Moms Letting Go private Facebook group, or both. You can share the print version, but I'd love to hear you say it out loud. The more moms we inspire with our courage, the more we will have on our team.

Notes from the All-Mighty Mom Tribe

Brooke

I want to have a story or two in Michelle's book, be able to speak about the parts I've written, help other moms into recovery, and share my experience, strength, and hope with those who continue to struggle.

***

Lucretia

It's a big deal to help write this book and the screenplay. I can see how these efforts will help many moms. We are making dreams come true.

I want to share the red flags, what to look for if you suspect your child is using, and how to implement the self-care steps necessary for recovery. Giving tools of hope will help moms thrive, not just survive!

***

Teresa

The fact I found this group of amazing moms was a God thing. I wasn't looking; I happened upon it. The strength I gained and the things I learned in the past six months is all due to the support of these women and the faith in God we share. Even though my addicted loved one has not chosen recovery yet, I am okay. I have survived the chaos, the disappointment, the heartache, and tears. The roller coaster will no doubt continue, but I will choose not to ride. The love we have for our children is like no other. We can continue to love them while caring for ourselves.

My Boon has always been to feel peace in my life. I think I'm getting close. I have another Boon to help the homeless get back on their feet. Since my son is currently part of that community, wouldn't it be something if someday my son and I were able to help others together? I would also love to help other moms in need of support as they travel this very difficult journey.

Thank you, Michelle. I am grateful to you and the All-Mighty Moms!

DAY 30

Create Your Boon

Twenty years from now you will be more disappointed
by the things that you didn't do than by the ones you did do.
So throw off the bowlines. Sail away from the safe harbor.
Catch the trade winds in your sails. Explore. Dream.
Discover.

—Unknown

Many moms of addicted loved ones choose not to share their stories to keep their child's life private. They feel guilty telling their story because it implicates their child as less than perfect. And because society sometimes views addiction as a choice and a moral failure, moms keep quiet. They suffer alone.

When we hide, we harbor more stigma. If we really believe addiction is a disease, then we should want everyone to know so they could pray for our child. If our child had cancer, we would garner support from prayer warriors everywhere. We might create posters and fundraisers. We would spread the word, knowing that faith brings miracles. Why then, can't we be open about our child's mental health diagnosis or SUD?

Only when moms move past this stigma mindset and ask for support will this ministry take charge.

One day, our great-grandchildren will wonder why we allowed people with an SUD to sit in jails and prisons and oftentimes be treated inhumanely. They will say, "How could human beings treat others so poorly and sleep at night?" This equates to us looking back on slavery or the Holocaust, and thinking, *How could anyone allow this to happen?*

Please don't misunderstand. I don't believe criminals should be allowed to do what they want, but when a person has a mental health disorder and an SUD, they need a plan for medical treatment. No one has ever been successful in punishing the pain out of these people. Most have been born into bad circumstances, endured trauma, or both. Incarceration isn't the solution. In many cases, it adds to the problem.

If you still have reservations about creating your Boon because of what others will think, let me set you straight. No one pays attention to what you do because most people spend their time focusing on themselves. If you become passionate about your Boon and you share it, others will notice.

If you get hacked, it doesn't serve you well. It might keep you safe and small, and that's okay if you aspire to safety and obscurity, but I know you're capable of leaving a bigger legacy.

As an *All-Mighty Mom on Fire* who understands unhackability, you have the power to create your Boon.

What If You Still Don't Have a Boon

If you find yourself stuck, not sure how to find your Boon, ask your friends and family what talents they see in you. Read the Bible. Ask God for clarification. Find an online assessment to help you define your spiritual gifts. And above all else, attend a local meeting or join our online group.

To get started with your imperfect action, assess the needs of your group. How can you serve? Start small. If time or money restraints freeze you, try volunteering at a church function or a substance use treatment center in your area. Consider contacting a homeless shelter. Can you prepare dinner one night? Plug in wherever you feel led. This doesn't need to be your big Boon. Each small act of service allows you to step out of your safe bubble and learn more about yourself. If we stay stuck in fear or lies, we will never heal, grow, or discover our gifts.

Boon Obstacles = Boon Opportunities

Before I started my book *Moms Letting Go Without Giving Up: Seven Steps to Self-Recovery* and the ministry to serve Moms of Addicted Loved Ones, I ran into many obstacles. I was exhausted raising two grandchildren. I drove them to and from school, which was not close to our home. At the time, I didn't know much about addiction and was angry at my son and daughter-in-law. Anxiety regarding their safety kept me up at night, and I was afraid anything I wrote would make me appear weak and my son appear like a failure. Fear held me back. What if I gave moms hope only to discover one of their children had overdosed? Did I have the time or energy to add another thing to my schedule? Could I learn enough technology to make connections and minister to moms? Plus, I didn't want to take time away from my husband; he had just retired.

But I learned obstacles can lead to opportunities.

Obstacles can serve as clues for achieving our Boon. We see more clearly when we change perspective. Instead of saying, "I'm too angry, tired, and afraid right now," I said, "I need to learn about addiction because at least a million other moms need to learn too."

Next, I thought, *if this is a calling from God, my lack of perfection doesn't matter. God will provide the time, the resources, and the knowledge. This will be an opportunity to grow. I don't have to do everything myself because I'm not alone. He walks with me, opening the doors, and helping me grow my knowledge to help others.*

How others see me isn't important. What matters is seeing myself as God sees me and knowing who to follow. It's about lives—lives that matter.

Let me show you how my specific obstacles became opportunities:

I was exhausted because I was raising two grandchildren.	• I realized I had an opportunity to exercise more and found more Energy.
I drove them to and from school because the school wasn't close to our home.	• We moved into a home that required less work and was closer to the schools.
I didn't know much about addiction.	• I took classes and became certified in addiction endeavors.
I was angry at my son and daughter-in-law.	• I learned their addiction wasn't a personal attack against me. It was a disease. In that shift, I was able to love my son and daughter-in-law.
I was afraid they would die.	• My faith grew as I realized we are all going to die, and God is in control. I took the time to grow a relationship with Him.

I was afraid to write something that might make me look weak.	•	Vulnerability gives me the opportunity to show others they're not alone.
I was afraid I would give moms hope only to discover that one of their children had overdosed.	•	This fear gave me the opportunity to reinforce the truth that I am not God. We all need hope.
I was afraid I didn't have the time or the energy to do one more thing.	•	I'm learning how to time-manage and do the things I love.
I didn't want to take time away from my husband in retirement.	•	I learned how to minister on the go. We can go wherever we want when we want. He is my greatest strength and supporter.
I didn't think I could learn online technology and make connections to build a brand that ministers to moms.	•	This ministry has given me the opportunity to learn how to podcast and form a private Facebook group that serves more than 1,800 moms. I can now navigate Instagram, Zoom, Google Docs, Anchor Podcasts, StreamYard, and Scrivener. And in the process, I gained confidence as I recognized it's not about me. It's about my message and the moms who need me. God counts on me to serve in this way, so He's helping this old lady learn new tricks every day.

If I hadn't been the mom of a child with an SUD, I wouldn't be committed to helping you on your journey. I wouldn't be here trying to empower one million moms. Philippians 4:13 is one of my favorite verses: "I can do all things through Christ, who strengthens me" (NRSV).

CLOSE YOUR GAP DAY 30: CREATE YOUR BOON

It's time to get into flow. Find your best way to feel inspiration and do some deep reflection in a quiet place. Turn your phone and computer notifications off and write. Don't judge or edit your words but don't think small. Go for big and bold. Use your imagination; the sky's the limit.

List Your Boon Obstacles—What keeps stopping you from starting?

_____

_____

_____

_____

Now, turn each obstacle into an opportunity. Ask yourself, "What could I do if I knew I couldn't fail? What if I believed my idea is a calling from God?" List clear productive actions you need to take.

List Your Boon Opportunities

_____

_____

_____

_____

Your Next Best Step

Your next step is turning your list of obstacles into opportunities. If you need help, we're here for you. Our Tribe and community exist to support you and set you on fire in your purpose. You'll find us here: HavocToHope.com

When you join our movement, you find sisters you never knew you had. Alone, we can make a difference, but together we can move mountains. I hope

> Sisterly love is one of the few boons in this life.
> **—Jane Bowles**

you'll join us in this crusade. I promise, you and your child are worth the fight.

One Simple Request

Now that you've discovered unhackability, please share this message with other moms. Spread the word. We need more All-Mighty Moms on fire to stop this epidemic, women who will work hard on their recovery so they can bring more change to our communities.

If you'd like to facilitate this thirty-day program in your community, I invite you to become a certified Unhackable Mom of an Addicted Loved One coach. To get details, reach out to me at Michelle@MichelleWeidenbenner.com.

If you'd like to continue studying this content, you can take the course at HavocToHope.com. You have the option to work alone or with one of our certified coaches.

We want to grow this in communities across the world. We can't wait to meet you and hear your Boon.

Notes from the All-Mighty Mom Tribe

This week I asked the Tribe two questions:

1. What would you do if you knew you couldn't fail?
2. Would you treat your idea differently if you knew it was from God?

I became emotional as I listened to their responses because I saw hope. I saw a glimpse of my own goal—helping moms recover so they can serve in this addiction epidemic space.

Marianne

I would want to change the recovery process. A twenty-eight-day inpatient treatment is not a program. I know insurance companies like to take the cheap and easy route, but honestly, no serious addict can recover in that time. I don't see how it can keep costs down in the long term. My son has been in rehab repeatedly. That costs a lot of money. Why not make the minimum commitment three months? With all the wasted money and time and the inadequacy of the programs, it's a miracle anyone ever finds successful recovery through them. If I knew I wouldn't fail, I would want to move the needle on that.

***

Lucretia

God will have to give me a whole lot more energy because I want to speak to women. I want a platform to convince women who have an addicted loved one they can change. The addiction epidemic is growing, and these women need help. They need to recognize the times they keep their children from accepting the consequences of their behavior—no matter how old their children are. Moms need to try something different. I've been talking to one woman back and forth and coaching her. It's exhausting. I need more energy. I would love to speak to a group of moms who want to change and understand the need for it. In less than a year, I've already seen how the choices of the moms in our group make a difference in the outcomes of our children.

***

Dawn

If I knew I wouldn't fail, I would set forth to find a cure for addiction, schizophrenia, and all the mental health disorders. A much younger me would build a respite village, a place women could go for a weekend, or a week, to clear their heads, get right with God, and get away.

I tried so hard to find a women's retreat, someplace I could go and be alone. After much searching, I found a place. It was the most relaxing, wonderful week. Anytime I want to return there mentally, I do, and it calms me. My kids gifted me this respite. I told them this was the gift that keeps on giving.

I anticipated working on my communication skills. I read self-help books and scheduled workshops to help me help Preston with his addiction; however, when I got there and looked around, I canceled my workshops—canceled them all. Instead, I sat at the beach, read books, went out to eat, rode my bicycle to the state park about ten miles away, and went looking for sharks' teeth on the beach. I got up early, just as the sun rose, so I could be the first person on the beach. I stopped to talk to people walking their dogs.

If I had the money, I would build a place on the beach or in the mountains where moms could come anytime they needed to escape.

***

My prayer is that each one of these women who have shared their vision in this Day will realize they can achieve what they want despite their perceived limitations. All it takes is an idea and trust that God will lead each little step from there.

APPENDICES

APPENDIX A
Motivational Interviewing

I learned about The Center for Motivation & Change (CMC) when I read the book *Beyond Addiction: How Science and Kindness Help People Change* by Jeffrey Foote, PhD.

Dr. Foote is the founder of CMC, a group of dedicated clinicians and researchers who rely on science and kindness to help people change. They employ respectful, flexible, evidence-based approaches to address substance use and compulsive behavior problems as well as other mental health issues, including trauma.

Motivational Interviewing (MI) is a collaborative conversation to strengthen a person's own motivation for and commitment to change. Though not therapists or scientists, moms are motivated to learn how to communicate more effectively. If we want to encourage change in our addicted children, it's imperative to learn how to listen better, have healthy conversations, and learn about change talk. This link gives more information on MI: Bit.ly/3FZ7yvD.

Some therapists don't recommend moms try this technique because we're too emotionally entrenched in our children's lives. I wanted to show you this resource so you could see the methods many rehabilitation centers and therapists use when they work with your children. We need to work with and listen to the professionals, and it can help us to understand some of their tools.

So often moms give up when their children succumb to addiction. They give their children to God and cut them out of their lives because they feel like they've tried everything and nothing has worked. They use the "let go and let God" approach. I understand. I operated in this place once, but I decided to avoid having regrets. I needed to educate myself on what I could do—not what I couldn't do. If my son died of an accidental overdose, I wanted to know I tried everything.

I encourage you to learn more about change talk and how you can develop better listening skills with your loved ones. It takes practice as well as courage and patience not to engage our negative emotions. It's not easy to meet our loved ones where they are even when we disagree. Even with a lot of work, we might never master this skill.

My purpose for mentioning MI here is to encourage you to learn more. I don't teach MI, but I take classes to practice and practice with moms in our support group. For more information on the Center for Motivation and Change, you can visit here: motivationandchange.com

I developed my own simple acronym to help you learn to listen better; you'll find it in Appendix B. But keep learning about MI. Don't get discouraged if you don't understand. Keep trying. Your children are worth your fight.

APPENDIX B
The BLESS *Method of Listening Using the* PEACE *Way*

Humans need to feel heard and understood. When we feel like no one cares about our point of view, we can become lonely, sad, withdrawn, frustrated, and angry. When our addicted loved ones feel judged, belittled, or like no one hears, it often triggers them to use again.

We can't control their actions, but we can learn how to communicate our care. We have one goal—to have no regrets should something happen to them or us. New strategies can help.

When you want to intentionally listen to your loved one, and he is coherent enough to have a conversation, using this technique can help. But getting good takes practice.

The Bless Method

Be Calm
Listen Better (PEACE way)
Empower your Child
Stay in your Lane
Short—Keep it Short

- **Be Calm.** Some say, "Hold your calm." This might be the most difficult step, so if you feel you're not in a good place emotionally to stay calm, it's better to wait until you've practiced this method with others—maybe in a support group or with your therapist.
- **Listen the PEACE Way.** I'll expand on this below.
- **Empower.** Empower your loved one to handle his problem. Ask, "What are your options?" and "What will you do?"
- **Stay in My Lane.** It's important to know your values so you stay within your boundaries and remain true to who you are and what you believe. If you're married, it's important to honor your spouse's values and boundaries too. It's easy to get distracted and interject an opinion in these conversations, so staying in our lane helps us focus on our goal. If we want to help our loved one feel seen and heard, it's imperative we stay committed to this practice.
- **Short.** Less is always better. If I say too much and feel like I'm starting to sound like a Lecture Queen, it's my cue to stop talking and listen more. Ask open-ended questions because they prompt them to talk more.

Listen the PEACE Way

Paraphrase
Emotion
Affirm
Consent
Empathy

- **Paraphrase** what your child says to you. Paraphrasing expresses the meaning of the speaker using different but similar words. This will help your child hear what he said. You can say, "Here's what I think you said _____. Did I get that right?" Paraphrasing also gives your child a chance to reword his statement or confirm that you heard him right.

- **Emotion.** Share the emotion you feel about his statement. "I feel <u>sad</u> (insert your emotion) that you're _____." If you experience anger, dig deeper into what emotion came before your anger. Did you feel frustration, grief, disappointment, guilt? Your loved one will probably react defensively to anger, and that won't help your relationship or provide a positive communication experience. Expressing the feeling you had that caused the anger will help defuse the situation; however, I highly recommend you talk to your therapist about your anger. If you can't come up with another emotion, skip this, and move to the next step.

- Alternately, you can mention his emotion. One example might be, "You sound frustrated." Noticing his emotion will help him feel validated, which is a part of our next step.

- **Affirm.** Affirming someone helps them feel heard. When we validate their feelings, we tell them we believe what they said. Affirming them as a person does not tell them we agree, only that we heard what they said.

- **Consent.** Moms often want to make suggestions but rarely ask permission. When we ask for consent to give a suggestion, we give the other person the choice to say yes or no. This shows respect. Ask, "Can I make a suggestion?" If they say, "No," then don't give your suggestion. If they give you permission, give your suggestion without lecturing.

- **Empathy.** It's okay to show our loved one empathy, as long as it doesn't lead to manipulation. If our loved one knows that when we're empathetic, we give them something they need to continue using, they will play that card. We must stay empathetic without enabling. Empathy shows you understand their plight, not that you pity them or want to help them fix their problem. You'll find a few examples of ways to show empathy below. Many can also give your loved one affirmation.

  - Thank you for sharing that with me.
  - Thank you for holding your calm.
  - I appreciate your patience.
  - What would be the best-case scenario for you?
  - Tell me more.
  - I wish you didn't have to go through this.
  - You must feel hopeless.
  - That must have hurt.
  - That must make you feel insecure.
  - That sounds frightening.
  - I can see why you're upset.
  - I see.

- What I admire most about what you're telling me is _____.
- You're in a tough spot.

An example of an exchange using the PEACE way.

CHILD: I lost my job.

MOM: You lost your job. (Paraphrase. No sarcasm or anger.)

CHILD: Yeah, I came in late. Stupid alarm didn't go off.

MOM: You sound upset. (Emotion)

CHILD: Hell yes, I'm pissed. I needed that job.

MOM: You gave them a lot of hours. I'm sure they'll miss you. (Affirm)

CHILD: I don't know what to do now.

MOM: Can I make a suggestion? (Consent)

CHILD: As long as you don't say, *I told you so.*

MOM: I heard that _____ is hiring. Maybe you could apply there. (Pat his hand or give his arm a squeeze.) Rejection never feels good. I'm sorry. (Empathy)

Another example:

CHILD: My cell phone broke.

MOM: Oh, your iPhone broke. (Paraphrase.)

CHILD: How am I supposed to get a job if nobody can get a hold of me?

MOM: I don't know. You sound frustrated. (Emotion.)

CHILD: Hell yes, I am. I'm not going to be able to pay you back or help with the kids' support this month.

MOM: Not being able to help hurts. (Affirm.)

CHILD: What am I going to do now?

MOM: Can I make a suggestion? (Consent.)

CHILD: No. Not unless you're going to give me the money for a new one.

MOM: No, remember the last time I helped I said it would be my last time? It's a new boundary, but it's one I'm going to stick to. This is tough for you, but I'm confident you're going to find the resources. I'll pray something changes for you. (Empathy.)

Here are examples of what we don't say. (But might have thought, said, or done.)

- Let me take care of that for you.
- Those idiots.
- Of course, you lost your job. You were late too many times.
- Maybe if you quit partying the night before, you'd make it on time.
- That's what you get.
- How are you going to pay your bills now?
- That was stupid.
- You're such an idiot.
- Don't ask me for more money.

When we rescue our children from their poor choices or the consequences of them, we rob them of their journey and what they learn along the way. On the other hand, when we belittle them or respond negatively, we confirm the feelings that drive them to use.

Sometimes it's our journey through life that launches us into our purpose.

Where there is pain, there is purpose. Robbing someone of their journey takes away their purpose.

APPENDIX C

Suggested Reading

For Parents of Addicted Loved Ones

A Second Chance: For You, for Me, and for the Rest of Us by Catherine Hoke

Beyond Addiction: How Science and Kindness Help People Change by Jeffrey Foote, PhD, Carrie Wilkens, PhD, and Nicole Kosanke, PhD, with Stephanie Higgs

Boundaries by Dr. Henry Cloud and Dr. John Townsend

Get Your Loved One Sober: Alternative to Nagging, Pleading, and Threatening by Robert J. Meyers

If You Love Me: A Mother's Journey Through Her Daughter's Addiction by Maureen Cavanaugh

In the Realm of Hungry Ghosts: Close Encounters with Addiction by Gabor Mate, MD

Jagged Little Edges by Lorelie Rozzano

Moms Letting Go Without Giving Up: Seven Steps to Self-Recovery by Michelle Weidenbenner.

Nonviolent Communication: A Language of Compassion by Marshall Rosenberg

Tending Dandelions: Honest Meditations for Mothers with Addicted Children (Just Dandy) by Sandra Swenson.

The Body Keeps the Score: Brain, Mind, and Body in the Healing of Trauma by Bessel van der Kolk, MD

The Joey Song: A Mother's Story of Her Son's Addiction by Sandra Swenson.

The Four Seasons of Recovery for Parents of Alcoholics and Addicts by Michael Speakman

Understanding and Helping an Addict (and Keeping Your Sanity) by Andrew Proulx, MD

Unhooked: How to Help an Addicted Loved One Recover by Jason Coombs

For Addicted Loved Ones

Celebrate Recovery 365 Daily Devotional: Healing from Hurts, Habits, and Hang-ups by John Baker

From Dope to Hope: A Man in Recovery by Tim Ryan

From Prison to Purpose by Jimmy McGill

If Not You, Then Who? Harness Your Strengths to Shift from Addiction to Abundance by Jesse Harless

Quitting to Win by Crystal Waltman

YouTube Channel

Put the Shovel Down, Amber Hollingsworth. https://www.youtube.com/channel/UCT8PE1v0xFR9zLXOijxM6hg

Podcast Recommendations

Heart of the Matter: Partnership to End Addiction with Elizabeth Vargas—https://podcasts.apple.com/us/podcast/heart-of-the-matter/id1534813640

Love Over Addiction—https://loveoveraddiction.com/podcast/

Moms Letting Go Without Giving Up with Michelle Weidenbenner—https://anchor.fm/michelle515

The Addiction Podcast| Point of No Return with Jonie Sigal—https://theaddictionpodcast.com

Unlocking Us with Brené Brown—https://brenebrown.com/podcast-show/unlocking-us

APPENDIX D
Breaking the Stigma with Proper Language

Say This	Not this
Person with a substance abuse disorder (SUD)	Addict, junkie, frequent-flyer, drug abuser
Person with alcohol use disorder	Alcoholic, drunk
Person in recovery or long-term recovery	Former addict, alcoholic, ex-addict
Person who previously used drugs	Reformed addict
Medication is a treatment tool	Medication is a crutch; one drug instead of another
Use; misuse; other than prescribed	Drug abuse

Opioid Agonist therapy; Pharmacotherapy; addiction medication, medication for a substance use disorder, medication for opioid use disorder (MOUD)	Opioid substitution replacement therapy; Medicated Assisted Treatment (MAT)
For toxicology screen results: testing negative	Clean
For non-toxicology purposes: Being in remission/recovery, abstinent from drugs; not drinking or taking drugs; not currently or actively using drugs	Clean
For toxicology screen results: testing positive	Dirty
For non-toxicology purposes: Person who uses drugs	Dirty
Baby born to mother who used drugs while pregnant; baby with signs of withdrawal from prenatal drug exposure; baby with neonatal opioid withdrawal/neonatal abstinence syndrome; newborn exposed to substances	Addicted baby
Substance use disorder; drug addiction	Habit
Drug poisoning	Drug overdose

For prescription medications: Misuse; used other than prescribed; For illicit drugs: Use	Abuse
Living with a substance use disorder	Battling/suffering from an addiction
Person arrested for a drug violation	Drug offender
Choose not to at this time	Non-compliant
Positive, negative, substance-free drug screen	Dirty drug screen
Reoccurrence of symptoms	Relapsed
Ambivalence	Denial
Protecting	Enabling
Loving well	Tough love
Pro-dependent	Co-dependent

Acknowledgments

My Family: Dave, Ryan and Angelika, Liza and Greg, Olivia and Cameron, and my grandchildren: Alanna, Addison, Patrick, and Claire. Thank you for understanding my passion for writing and supporting my efforts. I'm blessed by each one of you.

The All-Mighty Mom Tribe: Sandy Carmichael, Lucretia Renee Talley, Lily, Brooke Whitehead, Darra, Colleen, Carol, Angel, Dawn, Marianne, Teresa, Robin, Karen, and Lori.

Thank you for trusting me on your recovery journey. You helped me see how important it is to continue my *Boon* path to empower one million moms of addicted loved ones into recovery. You showed me what is possible when women come together to heal. You taught me more than I ever imagined possible. You strengthened my faith and affirmed my purpose. I am a better person because of each one of you.

Endnotes

1   Jesse C. Baumgartner and David C. Radley, "The Drug Overdose Toll in 2020 and Near-Term Actions for Addressing it," *The Commonwealth Fun,* August 16, 2021, https://www.commonwealthfund.org/blog/2021/drug-overdose-toll-2020-and-near-term-actions-addressing-it.

2   Michael Winnick, "Putting a Finger on our Phone Obsession," *Dscout*, Accessed April 8, 2020, https://blog.dscout.com/mobile-touches.

3   Vanessa Loder, "Why Multi-Tasking Is Worse Than Marijuana for Your IQ." *Forbes Magazine,* July 16, 2014.

4   "How to Watch Netflix on TV," *Reel In Reel*, March 29, 2020, https://www.reelnreel.com/watch-netflix-on-tv.

5   Louise Story, "Anywhere the Eye Can See, It's Likely to See an Ad." *The New York Times*, January 15, 2007, https://www.nytimes.com/2007/01/15/business/media/15everywhere.html.

6   Susan S. Land, "Mindless Autopilot' Drives People to Dramatically Underestimate How Many Daily Food Decisions They Make, Cornell

Study Finds," *Cornell Chronicle*, December 22, 2006, https://news.cornell.edu/stories/2006/12/ mindless-autopilot-drives-people-underestimate-food-decisions.

7   "Facts and Statistics," *Anxiety & Depression Association of America*, Accessed November 24, 2021, https://adaa.org/ understanding-anxiety/facts-statistics.

8   "Drug overdoses surged amid COVID lockdowns; more deaths in one year than ever before," November 17, 2021, https://www.usatoday.com/story/news/ health/2021/11/17/overdose-deaths-soar-record-level-ami d-pandemic-rise-fentanyl/8629870002.

9   James O. Prochaska, John C. Norcross, Carlo C. DiClemente, *Changing for Good: A Revolutionary Six-Stage Program for Overcoming Bad Habits and Moving Your Life Positively Forward* (New York: Quill-Harper Collins, 1994).

10 Kary Oberbrunner, *Unhackable: Closing the Gap Between Dreaming and Doing* (Powell, OH: Author Academy Elite, 2020).

11 Thomas Suddendorf, et al, "Mental Time Travel and the Shaping of the Human Mind," *National Center for Biotechnology Information*, May 2009, https://www.ncbi.nlm. nih.gov/pmc/articles/PMC2666704.

12 Joel Osteen, *Your Best Life Now* (Nashville: Hachette-FaithWords, 2014).

13 Cat Hoke, "The Power of Second Chances," *TEDx San Francisco*, November 3, 2017, https://youtu.be/ f4J1pgxYTww.

14 Hustle 2.0, A Self-Directed, In-cell Study Program for Incarcerated People, https://hustle20.com.

15 "Golden Buzzer: Nightbirde's Original Song Makes Simon Cowell Emotional," *America's Got Talent* June 8, 2021, https://www.youtube.com/watch?v=CZJvBfoHDk0.

16 "Seven Encouraging Nightbirde. Quotes," *Hope Has Arrived, Finding Hope, Strength, & Peace Against Cancer,* https://www. hopehasarrived.com/seven-encouraging-nightbirde-quotes.

17 Jane Marczewski, "Room For Air," *Nightbirde.co,/* May 3, 2021. https://www.nightbirde.co/blog.

18 Terry Small, "Brain Bulletin #47—The Science of Hope," *TerrySmall.com,* https://www.terrysmall.com/blog/ brain-bulletin-47-the-science-of-hope.

19 Amanda Enayati, "How Hope can Help You Heal," *CNN Health,* April 11, 2013, https://www.cnn.com/2013/04/11/ health/hope-healing-enayati/index.html.

20 Amanda Loudin, "The Fastest Growing Sport You've Never Heard Of," *NBCNews.com*, April 21, 2019, https://www.nbcnews.com/better/ lifestyle/pickleball-fastest-growing-sport-you-v e-never-heard-ncna992106.

21 Crystal Waltman, *Quitting to Win* (AAE: Powel, OH, 2020).

22 Napoleon Hill, *Think and Grow Rich* (Shippensburg, PA: Sound Wisdom, 1937).

23 Dr. Lee Angle, The Bright Light is Too Bright/Autism and Neurodevelopmental, October 28, 2021. https:// cityscoop.us/fortmyersfl-chiropractic/2021/10/28/ fort-myers-fl-the-bright-light-is-too-bright-autism-and-ne urodevelopmental.

24 Agarwal, Pragya. "Understanding Unconscious Bias," *Short Wave,* July 14, 2020, www.npr.org/2020/07/14/891140598/ understanding-unconscious.

25 Dace Radparvar, "Neurons that fire together, wire together." *Holstee.* Accessed June 25, 2020, https://www.holstee.com/blogs/mindful-matter/ neurons-that-fire-together-wire-together.

26 Vince Gill, "Go Rest High on That Mountain," *When Love Finds You*, MCA Nashville, August 28, 1995.

27 Paul Brian, "Constant Complaining is Bad for your Health and Rewires Your Brain," *Ideapod*, December 2020, www.ideapod.com/constant-complaining-is-bad-for-your-health.

28 Mike Oppland, "8 Ways to Create Flow According to Mihaly Csikszentmihalyi," *Positive Psychology*, February 15, 2021, https://positivepsychology.com/mihaly-csikszentmihalyi-father-of-flow.

29 Kimberly Holland, "What you Should Know about the Stages of Grief," *Healthline*, September 25, 2018, https://www.healthline.com/health/stages-of-grief.

30 Monica McGoldrick, "Genogram Video 2020," *Multicultural Family Institute,* May 22, 2020, https://www.youtube.com/watch?v=PT0HnwZGTYU.

31 Dr. Travis Bradberry, "How Complaining Rewires Your Brain for Negativity," *TalentsmartEQ*, https://www.talentsmarteq.com/articles/How-Complaining-Rewires-Your-Brain-for-Negativity-2147446676-p-1.html.

32 "Brain and Addiction," *National Institute on Drug Abuse, Advancing Addiction Science*, https://teens.drugabuse.gov/drug-facts/brain-and-addiction#topic-2.

33 Dr. Aimie, "Adverse Childhood Experiences and Addiction to Excitement," *Trauma Healing Accelerated*, August 3, 2017, https://draimie.com/addiction-to-excitement.

34 "How many times did Edison fail in attempting to invent the light bulb?" *Uncommon Content*, May 13, 2015, http://uncommoncontent.blogspot.com/2015/05/how-many-times-did-edison-fail-in.html.

35 Kendra Cherry, "What Is Neuroplasticity?" *Very Well Mind*, February 3, 2021, https://www.verywellmind.com/what-is-brain-plasticity-2794886.

36 Sandra Swenson, *Tending Dandelions: Honest Meditations for Mothers with Addicted Children* (Center City, MN: Hazelden Publishing, 2017).

HUGS
Our Core Values

Hope Builders

Notices the efforts of others
Compassionate
Encourager
Kind
Sees the heart of others
Positive
Owns her junk
Contributor

U

Unhackable Moms of Addicted Loved Ones

Victor mindset
Balances boundaries
Copes with chaos
Listens without lecturing
Contributor
Seeks truth tellers

G

Grow Girls

Learner
Motivated to change
Overcomer
Genuine
Survivor
Coachable
Connector
Brainstormer

S

Servant-Hearted Sisters

Compassionate
Spiritual
Eagerly encourages others
Thinks of others and herself
Compassionate listener
Calm
Empathetic
Anticipates needs

You've read
Unhackable Moms of Addicted Loved Ones.
Now it's time to take the online course.

Unhackable
Course

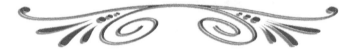

Closing the Gap Between Havoc and Hope

The 30-Day Program that helps you cope
with chaos, balance bold boundaries, and
listen without lecturing.

SCAN ME

Find out more at
HavocToHope.com

BECOME a CERTIFIED
Unhackable
Mom of an Addicted Loved One
COACH

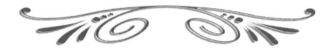

Get Paid to Help Moms
Close Their Gap Between Havoc and Hope

**Certified
Unhackable Mom
Coach, Speaker &
Trainter**

Learn More
HavocToHope.com

Moms Letting Go Without Giving Up

Seven Steps to Self-Recovery

Get Your Free Journal ebook.

SCAN ME

MomsLettingGo.com

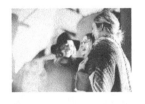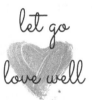

ALL
MIGHTY MOM
MEMBERSHIP

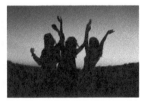

live fully

JOIN TODAY

JOIN our Support Group.
Healing happens in our community.

SCAN ME

Learn More:
HavocToHope.com

CPSIA information can be obtained
at www.ICGtesting.com
Printed in the USA
LVHW010730210622
721697LV00001B/3

9 781955 164092